Hypnic Headache

R. Silva-Néto • Dagny Holle-Lee

Hypnic Headache

Diagnosis and Treatment

Springer

R. Silva-Néto
Neurology
Federal University of the Parnaíba Delta
Parnaíba, Piauí, Brazil

Dagny Holle-Lee
Neurology
Essen University Hospital
Essen, Germany

ISBN 978-3-031-32262-4 ISBN 978-3-031-32263-1 (eBook)
https://doi.org/10.1007/978-3-031-32263-1

This Springer imprint is published by the registered company Springer Nature Switzerland AG
The registered company address is: Gewerbestrasse 11, 6330 Cham, Switzerland

To my dear parents, Osvaldo Carvalho e Silva (in memoriam) and Maria de Amorim Silva, for the countless efforts dedicated to my training and for the encouragement and affection with which they have always bestowed upon me.
To my wife and eternal companion, Adriana, and my son Lucas, for they understand my moments of absence, when I enter in the scientific world.
(R. Silva-Néto)

For my beloved son Winston, who kept me up many nights but never gave me a headache.
(Dagny Holle-Lee)

Foreword

Hypnic headache may be rare or occasional regarding prevalence, but definitely is a type of headache that specialists need to consider when dealing with sufferers on a common basis. The literature is scarce and mechanisms still uncertain, but chronobiological alterations or neurotransmitter dysfunctions, associated or not with sleep disturbances, seem to play a pathophysiological role.

There are probably many patients who have never received this diagnosis, despite suffering for a long time and having sought numerous professionals, during an average of 8 years, until a correct diagnosis is finally made. In this time, weird treatment attempts were commonly carried out. Caffeine, indomethacin, lithium, melatonin, and other drug options may be considered, but still with varied results.

The clinical presentation is not typical, but must be recognized, and the differential diagnosis is crucial. However, very few options of books and papers were available to provide the necessary knowledge. Through the years, since the initial descriptions of Neil Raskin, we were unable to encounter quality literature and again, when finding something, the usual modern plague of pharmaceutical industry interference.

This book, wrote by four hands, represents a turning point for hypnic headache education. It unveils a clear and objective approach, which most clinicians should remember when evaluating a headache with night presentation, even in children. It also discusses the paramount points of a diagnosis and reveals the fundaments for choosing the better treatment.

I have known Dr Silva-Néto for decades. He is the perfect example of a self-made physician. Struggling against all sorts of difficulties, Dr Silva-Néto is one of the most productive authors that I knew during my 35 years of Headache Medicine. No funding, industry money, grants of any kind and support for his considerable scientific achievements! It has been a great honor to perform, side by side with him, numerous studies dedicated exclusively to the field and not the profits.

Dr Holle-Lee is also a courageous pioneer in the study of hypnic headache. When most concentrate on the potentially profitable drug studies, she dedicated years and endurance to create knowledge on a less prevalent head pain. Her previous production in high-quality journals illustrates the challenges that hypnic headache posts to clarify its best approach and understanding.

This odd couple in science was united by pure serendipity but resulted in an immeasurable progress for all of us who face difficult patients with headache during the night. It is certain that we will enjoy and learn a lot with this unmissable book! It is a great pleasure to have this chance of highlighting the very good work of two luminaries of our field.

Headache Center of Rio
Rio de Janeiro, Brazil

Abouch V. Krymchantowski,

Preface

In 2001, during my headache internship in São Paulo (Brazil), I saw the first hypnic headache patient. In that year, only 52 cases of this disorder had been published worldwide; and in Brazil, only one case. Possibly, few Brazilian neurologists knew this diagnosis.

As a result of the experience acquired in the last 20 years about hypnic headache, I published several articles, such as case reports and case series, original articles and reviews, in addition to two book chapters. The description of 25 hypnic headache patients deserves to be highlighted, still the largest series of Brazilian cases; and two important reviews of cases published from 1988 to 2018: five in childhood and 343 in adults. In 2019, I wrote a book in Brazilian Portuguese entitled *Hypnic headache: Pains that come from sleep*.

Based on that experience, Dr. Holle-Lee and I decided to write ***Hypnic headache: Diagnosis and treatment***, a book with current knowledge on this subject. Briefly, we discussed historical aspects, epidemiology, clinical characteristics in children and adults, pathophysiology, differential diagnosis, and treatment of this rare form of headache.

We think this book will be useful to all doctors who care for headache patients, especially neurologists. Certainly, there will be an increase in accuracy in the hypnic headache diagnosis.

Parnaíba, Piauí, Brazil — R. Silva-Néto

Contents

About the Authors

Raimundo Silva-Néto, MD, PhD He received his medical degree from the Federal University of Piauí, in Teresina (Brazil), and completed a neurology residency at the Hospital of Restauração in Recife (Brazil). He completed a fellowship in headache at Headache Clinic Dr. Edgard Raffaelli Júnior, in São Paulo (Brazil), for one year. After completing his headache training, Dr. Silva-Néto completed his PhD in Neurology at Federal University of Pernambuco and his postdoctoral internship in Pharmaceutical Sciences at Federal University of Piauí. He is currently Professor of Neurology at Federal University of the Parnaíba Delta in Parnaíba (Brazil) and Member of the Brazilian Headache Society and International Headache Society.

Dagny Holle-Lee, MD, PhD Prof. Dagny Holle-Lee studied medicine in Mainz (Germany), Boston (USA), and Jerusalem (Israel). She completed her specialist training as a neurologist and cardiac specialist at the University Hospital in Essen (Germany). Since 2014, she has been head of the West German Headache and Vertigo Centre and is also senior physician in the neurological department. Her research interests are mainly in the pathophysiology and clinical presentation of headache and vertigo disorders. She is the author of numerous scientific articles and has also published several scientific and popular science books.

Abbreviations[1]

ABPM	ambulatory blood pressure monitoring
ACE	angiotensin converting enzyme
AMPA	a-amino-3-hydroxy-5-methyl-4-isoxazole propionic acid
ASA	acetylsalicylic acid
BC	before Christ
cAMP	cyclic adenosine monophosphate
CH	cluster headache
CHH	chronic hypnic headache
CNS	central nervous system
CPAP	continuous positive airway pressure
CSF	cerebrospinal fluid
CT	computed tomography
EEG	electroencephalogram
EHH	episodic hypnic headache
ESR	erythrocyte sedimentation rate
GABA	gamma-aminobutyric acid
GCA	giant cell arteritis
GH	growing hormone
HT	hydroxytryptamine
ICHD-2	International Classification of Headache Disorders, Second Edition
ICHD-3	International Classification of Headache Disorders, Third Edition
ICHD-3β	International Classification of Headache Disorders, Third Edition (beta version)
MAOIs	monoamine oxidase inhibitors
MOH	medication-overuse headache
MRI	magnetic resonance imaging
NDPH	new daily persistent headache
NSAIDs	nonsteroidal anti-inflammatory drugs

[1] Some acronyms were kept in their Anglo-Saxon forms, due to their universal meaning.

REM	rapid eye movement
SCN	suprachiasmatic nuclei
SSRIs	selective serotonin reuptake inhibitors
SUNA	short-lasting unilateral neuralgiform headache attacks with conjunctival injection and tearing
SUNCT	short-lasting unilateral neuralgiform headache attacks with cranial autonomic injection and tearing
TACs	trigeminal autonomic cephalalgias
TTH	tension-type headache
VAS	visual analogue scale

Chapter 1
Introduction

There is no pain that sleep can not overcome

Honoré de Balzac (1799–1850)

Over the past 30 years, there has been a huge advance in the study of headaches. Unusual forms of headaches have been described [1–4], new diagnostic criteria have been elaborated [5–8], some pathophysiological mechanisms have been elucidated and new drugs have been synthesized for treatment, both abortive [9–11] and prophylactic [12–14].

Among unusual headaches, there is hypnic headache, a rare form of headache that manifests itself in the elderly, during sleep [1]. Hypnic headache, as it is considered rare, is still little recognized and, therefore, underdiagnosed.

Although there are well-defined diagnostic criteria for hypnic headache in the current classification of headache [8], it seems that most doctors who care for the elderly with headache, such as neurologists, neurosurgeons, geriatricians, rheumatologists, ophthalmologists, otolaryngologists, and general practitioners are unaware of this diagnosis.

Usually, elderly people who have headache during sleep or when they wake up are diagnosed as having "migraine," even without a previous history of headache and without meeting the diagnostic criteria for migraine. In this way, the diagnosis will be wrong and, consequently, the treatment will also be.

This medical misinformation is due to the deficiency in the teaching of headache in most medical schools. In Brazil, for example, over a 6-year period, the medical student studies headache for around 2 h. After graduation, regardless of his/her specialty, this doctor will treat patients with headache, considered the main complaint of humanity.

For this reason, it is essential that doctors keep up to date, whether through participation in headache congresses or by reading good articles and specialized books. They will have more security in the care of headache patients and greater accuracy in their diagnoses if they were well informed.

R. Silva-Néto, D. Holle-Lee, *Hypnic Headache*,
https://doi.org/10.1007/978-3-031-32263-1_1

Since 1988, when the first cases were published, many researchers have studied hypnic headache. From 1988 to 2022, a total of 350 cases of hypnic headache have been published worldwide. One-third have been described in the American continent (81 in the USA and 35 in Brazil), 205 cases in Europe (more than 90% in 4 countries: Spain—99 cases, Italy—40 cases, Germany—30 cases, and France—23 cases), 27 in Asia, and 2 in Africa [15–18].

In addition to the case reports, reviews, and book chapters, two books were also published, one in Northern Ireland and the other in Brazil. Now a new book that aims to show, in a simple way, what is known about hypnic headache will be published. The preparation of this book was based on the review of all cases published in the last 34 years [15–17]. Several chapters of neurology books and more than 150 scientific articles on hypnic headache have been read.

The purpose of this book is obviously not to exhaust the subject, but to fill a gap in the medical literature. Further studies will be developed to improve medical knowledge regarding the understanding of the pathophysiology and treatment of this headache.

References

1. Raskin NH. The hypnic headache syndrome. Headache. 1988;28(8):534–6.
2. Negoro K, Morimatsu M, Ikuta N, Nogaki H. Benign hot bath-related headache. Headache. 2000;40(2):173–5.
3. Pareja JA, Caminero AB, Serra J, Barriga FJ, Barón M, Dobto JL, et al. Numular headache: a coin-shaped cephalgia. Neurology. 2002;58(11):1678–9.
4. Atkinson V, Lee L. An unusual case of an airplane headache. Headache. 2004;44(5):438–9.
5. Headache Classification Subcommittee of the International Headache Society. The international classification of headache disorders, 1st edition. Cephalalgia. 1988;8(7):10–96.
6. Headache Classification Subcommittee of the International Headache Society. The international classification of headache disorders, 2nd edition. Cephalalgia. 2004;24(1):8–160.
7. Headache classification Subcommittee of the International Headache Society. The international classification of headache disorders, 3rd edition (beta version). Cephalalgia. 2013;33(9):629–808.
8. Headache Classification Subcommittee of the International Headache Society. The international classification of headache disorders, 3rd edition. Cephalalgia. 2018;38(1):1–211.
9. Humphrey PP. The discovery of a new drug class for the acute treatment of migraine. Headache. 2007;47(1):10–9.
10. Humphrey PP. The discovery and development of the tryptans, a major therapeutic breakthrough. Headache. 2008;48(5):685–7.
11. Bigal ME, Walter S. Monoclonal antibodies for migraine: preventing calcitonin gene-related peptide activity. CNS Drugs. 2014;28(5):389–99.
12. Goadsby PJ, Reuter U, Hallström Y, Broessner G, Bonner JH, Zhang F, et al. A controlled trial of erenumab for episodic migraine. N Engl J Med. 2017;377(22):2123–32.
13. Hou M, Xing H, Cai Y, Li B, Wang X, Li P, et al. The effect and safety of monoclonal antibodies to calcitonin gene-related peptide and its receptor on migraine: a systematic review and meta-analysis. J Headache Pain. 2017;18(1):42.

14. Tepper S, Ashina M, Reuter U, Brandes JL, Dolezil D, Silberstein S, et al. Safety and efficacy of erenumab for preventive treatment of chronic migraine: a randomised, double blind, placebo-controlled phase 2 trial. Lancet Neurol. 2017;16(6):425–34.
15. Silva-Néto RP, Sousa-Santos PEM, Peres MFP. Hypnic headache: a review of 348 cases published from 1988 to 2018. J Neurol Sci. 2019;401:103–9.
16. Zhang Y, Wang C, Chen Y, Wang R, Lian Y. Hypnic headache with dopaminergic neuron dysfunction: new insight from a rare case. Pain Med. 2019;20(8):1639–42.
17. Kesserwani H. Hypnic headache responds to topiramate: a case report and a review of mechanisms of action of therapeutic agents. Cureus. 2021;13(3):13790.
18. Silva-Néto. Cefaleia hípnica: Dores que vem pelo sono. Nova Aliança: Teresina; 2019.

Chapter 2
Historical Aspects

In studying some seemingly new problems, we often make progress by reading the works of the great men of the past

Charles H. Mayo (1865–1939)

Hypnic Headache and Greek Mythology

In Ancient Greece, around 2000 BC, mythology was a way to guide the understanding of natural phenomena and other events that occurred without the intermediary of men. Greeks attributed each natural phenomenon to a different creature or God [1].

Gods were immortal and they were given all powers over nature, on which human survival depended. They had no supernatural characteristics but were portrayed in the likeness of man. They had human physical form; they had feelings and even the ability to feel pain [1].

Among these gods, there was Hypnos (Fig. 2.1), the god of sleep, responsible for the restorative rest of all terrestrial creatures, whether to recover wounds or even to replenish their energies. He was dressed in golden tones and had hair the same color. He had wings and always appeared with a flute on his lips, singing sweet songs that drove men to sleep. On his head, on the right side, there was a wing instead of an ear [2–6].

His parents were Erebus, the god of darkness, and Nyx, the goddess of the night. He had eight brothers and two sisters. They were: Thanatos, god of death; Ether, god of the sky; Hesperides, goddess of the afternoon; Philótes, god of friendship; Geras, god of old age; Momo, god of joy; Oizus, god of misery; Nemesis, goddess of vengeance; Kera, god of man's destiny in his final moments; and Moro, god of the share that each man will receive in life. Of all his brothers, the most important, without a doubt, was his twin Thanatos, the personification of death [2–6].

R. Silva-Néto, D. Holle-Lee, *Hypnic Headache*,
https://doi.org/10.1007/978-3-031-32263-1_2

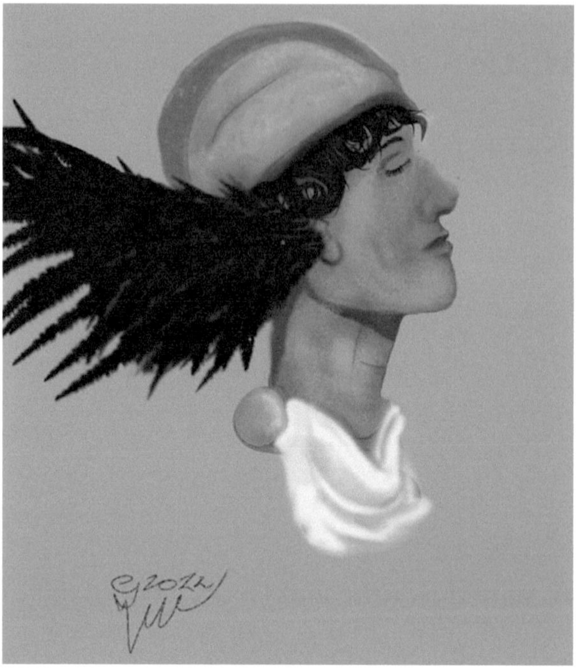

Fig. 2.1 Hypnos, the god of sleep (Drawing by Giordanno Santana Mazza, a medical student at the Federal University of the Parnaíba Delta, Brazil)

Hypnos had countless children, it is believed that more than a thousand, but only four of them stood out. A daughter, Fantasy, the goddess of delusion, responsible for distributing dreams to the awake; and three children, responsible for distributing dreams to those who slept. They were Morpheus, god of good dreams; Icelo, god of nightmares; and Phantasos, creator of inanimate objects that appear in dreams and remain in memory [2–6].

Hypnos is believed to have inhabited a palace built inside a large cave in the far west. Due to the depth of his kingdom, sunlight never penetrated there, so there was nothing to wake him up. In the middle of the palace, there was a bed surrounded by black curtains; in it, Hypnos could rest. At the entrance to the palace, his son Morpheus, the god of dreams, kept constant vigilance so that no one could wake him up.

From this mythological knowledge and, in allusion to the god Hypnos, the word "hypnic" (from the Greek "*hypnos*," sleep; and "*ic*," activity) was created, which refers to the phenomena that happen during sleep. On the other hand, the word headache or cephalalgia has long been part of the medical vocabulary. This expression, which is based on Greek etymology ("*kephalé*," head; and "*álgos*," pain) corresponds to pain that affects any region of the head, located or diffuse, from the eyes to the end of the hair implantation, in the nape region [1]. Therefore, hypnic headache is a headache that manifests itself during sleep.

Definition and Synonymy

Hypnic headache represents a rare type of recurrent primary headache, of short duration and without associated symptoms. It is characteristic of middle age and old age and always occurs during sleep, causing the patient to awaken [7]. For this reason, it became known previously as "clock headache" or "alarm clock headache." [8, 9]

The above definition induces the reader to think only of nocturnal awakening, but headache also occurs during daytime sleep awakening. There is a description of some cases of hypnic headache in which the pain appeared in the afternoon during naps, that is, in the short periods of time when the patient slept [10–14].

Even before the description of hypnic headache, this fact had already been reported in the 1970s, when American neurologists and specialists in sleep disorders, James D. Dexter (1935-) and Elliot D. Weitzman (1929–1983), observed the occurrence of headache during daytime naps [15].

The First Description

This headache was first described by the American neurologist Neil Hugh Raskin (1935-) in 1988, from a study of six patients seen between 1977 and 1986, of whom five were men; and one was a woman, aged 65–77 years. The headache woke them up and, in two of them, always after the dream, lasting 30–60 minutes. In three patients, the pain was throbbing. Only two of them reported migraine in the past, one with and one without aura. None of the patients had autonomic disorders that suggested cluster headache. The pain disappeared after using lithium carbonate, at a dose of 300–600 mg, at bedtime [16].

From this initial description made by Raskin, several case reports or case series on hypnic headache have been described in the literature, addressing their clinical and pathophysiological characteristics, in addition to the therapeutic response [8, 13, 14, 17–25].

The Diagnostic Criteria

In the years following the initial description of the hypnic headache, no diagnostic criteria were yet known. Despite this, in 1990, two new case reports were published, based on those from 1988 [9].

Until, in 1997, American neurologists Peter J. Goadsby and Richard B. Lipton proposed their first diagnostic criteria [26]. For these authors, in addition to the established diagnostic criteria, a rapid clinical response to lithium at bedtime would be expected (Table 2.1). This new headache should be included in item 4.7 of group

Table 2.1 Diagnostic criteria for hypnic headache suggested by Goadsby and Lipton (1997)

A. Headache occurs at least 15 times per month for at least 1 month.
B. Headache awaken patient from sleep.
C. Attacks duration of 5–60 minutes.
D. Pain is generalized or unilateral.
E. Pain not associated with autonomic features.
F. At least one of the following:
1. There is no suggestion of one of the disorders listed in groups 5–11.
2. Such a disorder is suggested but excluded by appropriate investigations.
3. Such a disorder is present but the first headache attacks do not occur in close temporal relation to the disorder.

Table 2.2 Diagnostic criteria for hypnic headache, suggested by Evers and Goadsby (2003)

A. Headache occurs at least 15 times per month for at least 1 month.
B. Headache awaken patient from sleep.
C. Usual attacks duration of 10–180 minutes.
D. Pain is not associated with cranial autonomic features that fulfill a diagnosis of group 3 (e.g., cluster headache and chronic paroxysmal hemicrania).
E. Patient should usually not have any of the following features associated with the headache:
1. Nausea.
2. Photophobia.
3. Phonophobia.
4. Aggravation of headache with routine physical activity.
F. At least one of the following:
1. There is no suggestion of one of the disorders listed in groups 5–11.
2. Such a disorder is suggested but excluded by appropriate investigations.
3. Such a disorder is present but the first headache attack does not occur in close temporal relation to the disorder.

4 (various headaches not associated with structural injury) of the 1988 headache classification [27].

From then on, several reports of hypnic headache began to be described worldwide. In 1997, eight new cases were published [28–30], including the first Brazilian case, described by neurologists Luiz Paulo Queiroz and Luiz Carlos Coral [29].

In 1999, Spanish neurologist Francisco Morales Asín published the first review on hypnic headache, with 39 cases reported to date. He described its clinical characteristics, pathophysiology, and treatment [31]. The second review was written in 2003, by American neurologists Stefan Evers and Peter J. Goadsby describing 71 cases up to that year [32]. These authors modified the diagnostic criteria for hypnic headache, making them a little more specific than the previous ones (Table 2.2).

In September 2014, a major review was published of the 255 cases of hypnic headache [33] described since 1988, up to that year, based on case reports and eight large series [8, 20–25, 34]. In June 2019, the most recent literature review on hypnic

Table 2.3 The 11 largest case series on hypnic headache published between 1988 and 2018

Authors	Country of origin	Sample	Publication reference
Manni et al.	Italy	10	Neurology 2004;62(8):1411–3
Mulero et al.	Spain	13	Rev Neurol 2012;54(3):129–36
Liang et al.	Taiwan	17	Cephalalgia 2008;28(3):209–15
Dodick et al.	USA	19	Cephalalgia 1998;18(3):152–6
Holle et al.	Germany	20	Cephalalgia 2010;30(12):1435–42
Donnet and Lantéri-Minet	France	22	Cephalalgia 2009;29(9):928–34
Jiménez-Caballero et al.	Spain	24	Rev Neurol 2012;54(6):332–6
Silva-Néto and Almeida	Brazil	25	J Neurol Sci 2014;338(1–2):166–8
Ruiz et al.	Spain	23	Headache 2015;55(1):167–73
Escudero Martínez et al.	Spain	10	Neurologia 2015;30(4):195–200
Tariq et al.	USA	40	Headache 2016;56(4):717–24

Source: Silva-Néto. Cefaleia hípnica: Dores que vem pelo sono. Nova Aliança: Teresina, 2019

Table 2.4 The nine major reviews on hypnic headache published from 1988 to 2018

Author(s)	Country of origin	Sample	Publication reference
Morales-Asín	Spain	39	Rev Soc Esp Dolor 1999;6(5):363–7
Evers and Goadsby	Germany	71	Neurology 2003:60(6):905–9
Evers and Goadsby	Germany	94	Practical Neurology 2005;5(3):144–9
Gil-Gouveia and Goadsby	Portugal	101	J Neurol 2007;254(5):646–54
Lisoto et al.	Italy	119	Headache Pain 2010;11(4):349–54
Lantéri-Minet and Donnet	France	154	Curr Pain Headache Rep 2010;14(4):309–15
Holle et al.	Germany	225	Cephalalgia 2013;33(16):1349–57
Liang and Wang	Taiwan	255	Cephalalgia 2014;34(10):795–805
Silva-Neto et al.	Brazil	348	J Neurol Sci 2019;401:103–9.

Source: Silva-Néto. Cefaleia hípnica: Dores que vem pelo sono. Nova Aliança: Teresina, 2019

headache was published, in which 348 patients (343 adults and 5 children) were described [35].

In the past 34 years, 11 large case series (≥10 patients per publication) have been published, totaling more than 200 patients (Table 2.3) [8, 17–25, 34], and nine major reviews on hypnic headache (Table 2.4) [31–33, 36–41].

Finally, in 2004, hypnic headache was included in the second edition of the International Classification of Headache Disorders (ICHD-2), in group 4.5 "Other primary headaches" (Table 2.5) [42].

In 2006, four Italian researchers (Roberto de Simone, Enrico Marano, Angelo Ranieri, and Vicenzo Bonavita) published an important study that resulted in the following contributions: expansion of the clinical spectrum of this headache, inclusion of clinical forms lasting more than 3 h, and expanding knowledge of therapeutic options [43].

Table 2.5 Diagnostics criteria for hypnic headache according to ICHD-2 (2004)

A. Dull headache fulfilling criteria B-D.
B. Develops only during sleep, and awakens patients.
C. At last two of the following characteristics:
1. Occurs >15 times per month.
2. Lasts ≥15 minutes after waking.
3. First occurs after the age of 50 years.
D. No autonomics symptoms and no more than one of nausea, photophobia, or phonophobia.
E. Not attributed to another disorder.

Table 2.6 Diagnostics criteria for hypnic headache according to ICHD-3β (2018)

A. Recurrent headache attacks fulfilling criteria B–E.
B. Developing only during sleep, and causing wakening.
C. Occurring on ≥10 days/month for >3 months.
D. Lasting from 15 minutes up to 4 hours after waking.
E. No cranial autonomic symptoms or restlessness.
F. Not better accounted for by another ICHD-3 diagnosis.

Table 2.7 ICHD-3 diagnostic criteria for probable hypnic headache

A. Recurring headache attacks fulfilling criteria B and C.
B. Developing only during sleep, and causing wakening.
C. Two only of the following:
1. Occurring on ≥10 days / month for >3 months.
2. Lasting from 15 minutes up to 4 hours after waking.
3. No cranial autonomic symptoms or restlessness.
D. Not fulfilling ICHD-3 criteria for any other headache disorders.
E. Not better accounted for by another ICHD-3 diagnosis.

In 2013, the third edition of the classification of headache was published, in its beta version, the ICHD-3β. In this classification, hypnic headache was included in group 4.9 and described as frequent recurrent headache attacks, which develop only during sleep, causing awakening, lasting more than 15 minutes and for up to 4 hours, without associated autonomic symptoms and not attributed to another pathology (Table 2.6) [43].

In January 2018, the third edition of the classification of headache was published in its final version [7]. There was no change from the previous classification, but the diagnostic criteria for the probable hypnic headache were included (Table 2.7).

Books on Hypnic Headache

Over the past 34 years, many researchers worldwide have extensively studied hypnic headache. In that time, more than a hundred articles, several book chapters, and two books were published.

The first book was published in Northern Ireland, in 2013, by neurologist Dr. Raeburn B. Forbes, with the title "Hypnic Headache – Your definitive guide." It was written in English, easy to read, and based on a review of all cases published up to that time. Dr. Forbes graduated in Medicine from the University of Dundee Medical School, in the city of Dundee (Scotland), in 1992 [44]. He currently works at the Apex Headache Clinic in Belfast, Northern Ireland [43].

The second book was published in Brazil, in 2019, by neurologist R. Silva-Néto, titled "Hypnic Headache – Pain that comes from sleep." It was written in Brazilian Portuguese and was based on a review of 348 published cases from 1988 to 2018 [35]. Dr. Silva-Néto graduated in Medicine from the Federal University of Piauí, in the city of Teresina (Brazil), in 1995. For the past 20 years, he has been dedicated to caring for headache patients. He is currently a professor of Neurology at the Federal University of the Parnaíba Delta, in Parnaíba (Brazil).

Turtle Headache

Headaches that occur on awakening are older than you think. In 1972, long before the hypnic headache was known, the American neurologist Gordon J. Gilbert described an unusual headache called turtle headache [45].

It is a bilateral headache that occurs only in the morning, upon awakening, when the patient pulls the blankets from the bed over his head or retracts his head under the blankets, like a turtle hiding under his shell [45, 46]. It is considered rare because there is little information and patients are not diagnosed.

Initially, this headache was characterized as a primary headache. A few years later, it was suggested that hipoxia was the underlying cause of this headache, when pulling the blanket over the head in an environment with less oxygen. Therefore, turtle headache should be considered symptomatic hypnic headache [47].

Unfortunately, there is little information about turtle headache and it is not always diagnosed. Possibly, many patients may suffer from turtle headache, as occurs with the underdiagnosis of hypnic headache. The frequency of this headache is unknown and no familial cases have been reported [46].

The diagnosis of turtle headache is based on the clinical history, as the patient will report that the headache occurs after awakening, and then he will try to go back to sleep by pulling the blanket over his head. Despite being recognized as a primary headache, neuroimaging tests should be performed to rule out secondary causes [46].

The pathophysiology of turtle headache is unknown because little data is available. In addition to hypoxia, it is believed that there are also hypothalamic changes.

There are studies that have demonstrated a possible link between hypoxia, migraine, and cluster headache [48].

Hypoxia is believed to play an important role in the pathophysiology of turtle headache because other headaches are associated with hypoxia. In cerebral vasodilation by hypoxia and in individuals who ascend to heights above 3000 meters, headache occurs. In addition, there are studies demonstrating that cortical spreading depression, present in the pathogenesis of migraine, is induced by hypoxia [49, 50].

In addition to hypoxia, it is suspected that these patients have changes in gray matter volume in the posterior hypothalamus, which is the biological clock of the human body. This hypothesis has not been proven in hypnic headache, but there are studies on the volume of the hypothalamus as a diagnostic biomarker of chronic migraine [46].

No studies have specifically looked at turtle headache. Despite these pains persisting for years, the prognosis appears to be good and there are no significant complications. In general, most patients get relief after treatment that is similar to that of hypnic headache (described in Chap. 9). However, the patient should be instructed to follow some non-pharmacological measures, such as avoid pulling the blanket over the head while in bed, have healthy sleep hygiene, and practice physical exercises to ensure adequate oxygenation.

References

1. Silva-Néto R. Cefaleias noturnas. In: Silva-Néto R, editor. Cefaleia – aspectos históricos e tópicos relevantes. Teresina: Halley; 2013. p. 139–44.
2. Swick TJ. The neurology of sleep. Neurol Clin. 2015;23(4):9671–89.
3. Bause GS. Hypnos, god of sleep. Anesthesiology. 2013;119(2):255.
4. Sleigh J. Disentangling Hypnos from his poppies. Anesthesiology. 2010;113(2):271–2.
5. Brandão JS. Dicionário Mítico-Etimológico da Mitologia Grega. Petrópolis: Vozes; 2008.
6. Gravitz MA, Gerton MI. Origins of the term hypnotism prior to braid. Am J Clin Hypn. 1984;27(2):107–10.
7. Headache Classification Subcommittee of the International Headache Society. The international classification of headache disorders, 3rd edition. Cephalalgia. 2018;38(1):1–211.
8. Dodick DW, Mosek AC, Campbell JK. The hypnic ('alarm clock') headache syndrome. Cephalalgia. 1998;18(3):152–6.
9. Newman LC, Lipton RB, Solomon S. Hypnic headaches. Headache. 1990;30(4):236.
10. Prakash S, Dahbi AS. Relapsing remitting hypnic headache responsive to indomethacin in an adolescent: a case report. J Headache Pain. 2008;9(6):393–5.
11. Dolso P, Merlino G, Fratticci L, Canesin R, Valiante G, Coccolo D, et al. Non-REM hypnic headache: a circadian disorder? A clinical and polysomnography. Cephalalgia. 2006;27(1):83–6.
12. Pinessi L, Rainero I, Cicolin A, Zibetti M, Gentile S, Mutani R. Hypnic headache syndrome: association of the attacks with REM sleep. Cephalalgia. 2003;23(2):150–4.
13. Ghiotto N, Sances G, Di Lorenzo G, Trucco M, Loi M, Sandrini G, et al. Report of eight new cases of hypnic headache and mini-review of the literature. Funct Neurol. 2002;17(4):211–9.
14. Pinto CAR, Fragoso YD, Souza Carvalho D, Gabbai AA. Hypnic headache syndrome: clinical aspects of eight patients in Brazil. Cephalalgia. 2002;22(10):824–7.

15. Dexter JD, Weitzman ED. The relationship of nocturnal headaches to sleep stage patterns. Neurology. 1970;20(5):513–8.
16. Raskin NH. The hypnic headache syndrome. Headache. 1988;28(8):534–6.
17. Tariq N, Estemalik E, Vij B, Kriegler JS, Tepper SJ, Stillman MJ. Long-term outcomes and clinical characteristics of hypnic headache syndrome: 40 patients series from a tertiary referral center. Headache. 2016;56(4):717–24.
18. Ruiz M, Mulero P, Pedraza MI, de la Cruz C, Rodríguez C, Muñoz I, et al. From wakefulness to sleep: migraine and hypnic headache association in a series of 23 patients. Headache. 2015;55(1):167–73.
19. Escudero Martínez I, González-Oria C, Bernal Sánchez-Arjona M, Jiménez Hernández MD. Description of series of 10 patients with hypnic headache: discussion of the diagnostic criteria. Neurologia. 2015;30(4):195–200.
20. Silva-Néto RP, Almeida KJ. Hypnic headache: a descriptive study of 25 new cases in Brazil. J Neurol Sci. 2014;338(1–2):166–8.
21. Mulero P, Guerrero-Peral AL, Cortijo E, Jabary NS, Herrero-Velázquez S, Miranda S, et al. Cefalea hípnica: características de una serie de 13 nuevos casos y propuesta de modificación de los criterios diagnósticos. Rev Neurol. 2012;54(3):129–36.
22. Jiménez-Caballero PE, Gámez-Leyva G, Gómez M, Casado-Naranjo I. Descripción de una serie de casos de cefalea hípnica. Diferenciación entre sexos Rev Neurol. 2012;54(6):332–6.
23. Holle D, Naegel S, Krebs S, Katsarava Z, Diener HC, Gaul C, et al. Clinical characteristics and therapeutic options in hypnic headache. Cephalalgia. 2010;30(12):1435–42.
24. Donnet A, Lantéri-Minet M. A consecutive series of 22 cases of hypnic headache in France. Cephalalgia. 2009;29(9):928–34.
25. Liang JF, Fuh JL, Yu HY, Hsu CY, Wang SJ. Clinical features, polysomnography and outcome in patients with hypnic headache. Cephalalgia. 2008;28(3):209–15.
26. Headache Classification Subcommittee of the International Headache Society. The international classification of headache disorders. Cephalalgia. 1988;8(7):10–96.
27. Goadsby PJ, Lipton RB. A review of paroxysmal hemicranias, SUNCT syndrome and other short-lasting headaches with autonomic feature, including new cases. Brain. 1997;120(1):193–209.
28. Gould JD, Silberstein SD. Unilateral hypnic headache: a case study. Neurology. 1997;49(6):1749–51.
29. Queiroz LP, Coral LC. The hypnic headache syndrome – a case report (Abstract). Proceedings of 8th Congress of the International Headache Society, 1997 Jun 10–14; Amsterdam, Germany. Cephalalgia. 1997;17(3):303.
30. Skobieranda FG, Lee TG, Solomon GD. The hypnic headache syndrome: six additional patients (Abstract). Proceedings of 8th congress of the international headache society, 1997 Jun 10-14; Amsterdam, Germany. Cephalalgia. 1997;17(3):304–5.
31. Morales F. Síndrome de cefalea hípnica. Revisión Rev Soc Esp Dolor. 1999;6(5):363–7.
32. Evers S, Goadsby PJ. Hypnic headache: clinical features, pathophysiology, and treatment. Neurology. 2003;60(6):905–9.
33. Liang JF, Wang SJ. Hypnic headache: a review of clinical features, therapeutic options and outcomes. Cephalalgia. 2014;34(10):795–805.
34. Manni R, Sances G, Terzaghi M, Ghiotto N, Nappi G. Hypnic headache: PSG evidence of both REM-and NREM-related attacks. Neurology. 2004;62(8):1411–3.
35. Silva-Néto RP, Sousa-Santos PEM, Peres MFP. Hypnic headache: a review of 348 cases published from 1988 to 2018. J Neurol Sci. 2019;401:103–9.
36. Holle D, Naegel S, Obermann M. Hypnic headache. Cephalalgia. 2013;33(16):1349–57.
37. Lisotto C, Rossi P, Tassorelli C, Ferrante E, Nappi G. Focus on therapy of hypnic headache. J Headache Pain. 2010;11(4):349–54.
38. Lanteri-Minet M, Donnet A. Hypnic headache. Curr Pain Headache Rep. 2010;14(4):309–15.
39. Gil-Gouveia R, Goadsby PJ. Secondary hypnic headache. J Neurol. 2007;254(5):646–54.
40. Evers S, Goadsby PJ. Hypnic headache. Pract Neurol. 2005;5(3):144–9.

41. Headache Classification Subcommittee of the International Headache Society. The international classification of headache disorders, 2nd edition. Cephalalgia. 2004;24(1):8–160.
42. De Simone R, Marano E, Ranieri A, Bonavita V. Hypnic headaches: an update. Neurol Sci. 2006;27(2):144–8.
43. Headache classification Subcommittee of the International Headache Society. The international classification of headache disorders, 3rd edition (beta version). Cephalalgia. 2013;33(9):629–808.
44. Forbes RB. Hypnic headache – your definitive guide. Northern Ireland: Forbes Neurology Services Ltd; 2013.
45. Gilbert GJ. Hypoxia and bedcovers. JAMA. 1972;221(10):1165–6.
46. Patel P, Prabhu A, Tadi P. Turtle headache. In: StatPearls [internet]. Treasure Island. Florida: StatPearls Publishing; 2022.
47. Gilbert GJ. Turtle headache. JAMA. 1982;248(8):921.
48. Britze J, Arngrim N, Schytz HW, Ashina M. Hypoxic mechanisms in primary headaches. Cephalalgia. 2017;37(4):372–84.
49. Carod-Artal FJ. High-altitude headache and acute mountain sickness. Neurologia. 2014;29(9):533–40.
50. Somjen GG, Aitken PG, Czéh GL, Herreras O, Jing J, Young JN. Mechanism of spreading depression: a review of recent findings and a hypothesis. Can J Physiol Pharmacol. 1992;70:248–54.

Chapter 3
Headaches Classification

Science progresses best when observations force us to change our preconceived ideas

Vera Rubin (1928–2016)

Introduction

Headache is the main complaint in neurology and its correct diagnosis requires, on the part of the doctor, knowledge of the diseases that can cause this symptom. For this, there is an international classification of headache, cranial neuralgia, and facial pain. Unfortunately, some doctors, for various reasons, ignore the diagnostic criteria contained in this classification.

According to the descriptions found in Egyptian papyri and other archaeological findings, we know that headache is an ancient complaint of humans [1, 2]. However, its study worldwide began, effectively, in the 1930s, with the American neurologist Harold George Wolff (1898–1962). He began to investigate its causes and to classify the different groups of headache [3–6]. In Latin America, the study of headache began with the Brazilian neurologist Edgard Raffaelli Júnior (1930–2006), in 1956 [4, 7, 8].

In 1962, the first headache classification developed by a group of American researchers (Arnold P. Friedman, Harold George Wolff, John Ruskin Graham, E. Charles Kunkle, Knox Finley, and Adrian Ostfeld) emerged [4, 9].Although this classification was genuinely American, it remained as a guideline for 26 years for those interested in headache worldwide.

In 1988, the first International Classification of Headaches, Cranial Neuralgias and Facial Pain was created, differing from the 1962 classification in that it includes operational diagnostic criteria for all headaches. In this classification, 12 major categories of headache were identified, divided into two large groups: primary headaches (categories 1–4) and secondary headaches (categories 5–12) [10].

R. Silva-Néto, D. Holle-Lee, *Hypnic Headache*,
https://doi.org/10.1007/978-3-031-32263-1_3

In 2004, the International Classification of Headache Disorders, Second Edition (ICHD-2) was published [11]; in 2013, the International Classification of Headache, Third Edition (beta version) (ICHD-3β) [12]; and in 2018, the International Classification of Headache, Third Edition (ICHD-3) [13], the most recent, expanded and revised classification, describing almost 300 different types of headache. ICHD-3 is divided into three parts: primary headaches, secondary headaches, and painful cranial neuropathies and other facial pain [12]. Its use is suggested in medical practice and clinical research.

Undoubtedly, the elaboration of an internationally accepted classification of headache was extremely important to standardize diagnoses, giving greater homogeneity to studies from the most diverse research centers.

In primary headaches, there is no structural injury, as the problem is purely biochemical. Routine examinations are normal. Primary headaches are usually diagnosed only by their clinical characteristics, such as time of onset, location, duration, frequency and intensity of attacks, associated symptoms, and triggering factors. So far, there is no subsidiary examination to diagnose a primary headache.

Primary headaches correspond to 90% of headaches. They are divided into four groups: migraine, tension-type headache, trigeminal autonomic cephalalgias, and other primary headache disorders [13]. In the fourth group, there are 10 different types of headaches: primary cough headache, primary exercise headache, primary headache associated with sexual activity, primary thunderclap headache, cold-stimulus headache, external-pressure headache, primary stabbing headache, nummular headache, hypnic headache, and new daily persistent headache. This classification is shown in Table 3.1.

On the other hand, secondary headaches (Table 3.2) are due to organic diseases. They cover a wide variety of headaches caused by the most diverse reasons, for example, head trauma, arteritis, cerebral venous thrombosis, intracerebral hematoma, aneurysm rupture, intracranial hypertension, exposure or withdrawal from any substance, systemic or intracranial infections, disorders of the eyes, ears, nose, sinuses, and teeth.

The third part of ICHD-3[13] consists of painful lesions of the cranial nerves, other facial pain, and other headache disorders as shown in Table 3.3.

Table 3.1 Primary headaches—Part I of ICHD-3 (groups 1–4)

1. Migraine.
- 1.1. Migraine without aura.
- 1.2. Migraine with aura.
- 1.3. Chronic migraine.
- 1.4. Complications of migraine.
- 1.5. Probable migraine.
- 1.6. Episodic syndromes that may be associated with migraine.

2. Tension-type headache.
- 2.1. Infrequent episodic tension-type headache.
- 2.2. Frequent episodic tension-type headache.
- 2.3. Chronic tension-type headache.
- 2.4. Probable tension-type headache.

3. Trigeminal autonomic cephalalgias.
- 3.1. Cluster headache.
- 3.2. Paroxysmal hemicrania.
- 3.3. Short-lasting unilateral neuralgiform headache attacks.
- 3.4. Hemicrania continua.
- 3.5. Probable trigeminal autonomic cephalalgia.

4. Other primary headache disorders.
- 4.1. Primary cough headache.
- 4.2. Primary exercise headache.
- 4.3. Primary headache associated with sexual activity.
- 4.4. Primary thunderclap headache.
- 4.5. Cold-stimulus headache.
- 4.6. External-pressure headache.
- 4.7. Primary stabbing headache.
- 4.8. Nummular headache.
- 4.9. Hypnic headache.
- 4.10. New daily persistent headache (NDPH).

Table 3.2 Secondary headaches—Part II of ICHD-3 (groups of 5–12)

5. Headache attributed to trauma or injury to the head and/or neck.
- 5.1. Acute headache attributed to traumatic injury to the head.
- 5.2. Persistent headache attributed to traumatic injury to the head.
- 5.3. Acute headache attributed to whiplash.
- 5.4. Persistent headache attributed to whiplash.
- 5.5. Acute headache attributed to craniotomy.
- 5.6. Persistent headache attributed to craniotomy.

6. Headache attributed to cranial and/or cervical vascular disorder.
- 6.1. Headache attributed to cerebral ischemic event.
- 6.2. Headache attributed to non-traumatic intracranial haemorrhage.
- 6.3. Headache attributed to unruptured vascular malformation.
- 6.4. Headache attributed to arteritis.
- 6.5. Headache attributed to cervical carotid or vertebral artery disorder.
- 6.6. Headache attributed to cranial venous disorder.
- 6.7. Headache attributed to other acute intracranial arterial disorder.
- 6.8. Headache and/or migraine-like aura attributed to chronic intracranial vasculopathy.
- 6.9. Headache attributed to pituitary apoplexy.

7. Headache attributed to non-vascular intracranial disorder.
- 7.1. Headache attributed to increased cerebrospinal fluid (CSF) pressure.
- 7.2. Headache attributed to low cerebrospinal fluid (CSF) pressure.
- 7.3. Headache attributed to non-infectious inflammatory intracranial disease.
- 7.4. Headache attributed to intracranial neoplasia.
- 7.5. Headache attributed to intrathecal injection.
- 7.6. Headache attributed to epileptic seizure.
- 7.7. Headache attributed to Chiari malformation type I (CM1).
- 7.8. Headache attributed to other non-vascular intracranial disorder.

8. Headache attributed to a substance or its withdrawal.
- 8.1. Headache attributed to use of or exposure to a substance.
- 8.2. Medication-overuse headache (MOH).
- 8.3. Headache attributed to substance withdrawal.

9. Headache attributed to infection.
- 9.1. Headache attributed to intracranial infection.
- 9.2. Headache attributed to systemic infection.

10. Headache attributed to disorder of homoeostasis.
- 10.1. Headache attributed to hypoxia and/or hypercapnia.
- 10.2. Dialysis headache.
- 10.3. Headache attributed to arterial hypertension.
- 10.4. Headache attributed to hypothyroidism.
- 10.5. Headache attributed to fasting.
- 10.6. Cardiac cephalalgia.
- 10.7. Headache attributed to other disorder of homoeostasis.

11. Headache or facial pain attributed to disorder of the cranium, neck, eyes, ears, nose, sinuses, teeth, mouth or other facial or cervical structure.
- 11.1. Headache attributed to disorder of cranial bone.
- 11.2. Headache attributed to disorder of the neck.
- 11.3. Headache attributed to disorder of the eyes.
- 11.4. Headache attributed to disorder of the ears.
- 11.5. Headache attributed to disorder of the nose or paranasal sinuses.
- 11.6. Headache attributed to disorder of the teeth.
- 11.7. Headache attributed to temporomandibular disorder (TMD).
- 11.8. Head or facial pain attributed to inflammation of the stylohyoid ligament.
- 11.9. Headache or facial pain attributed to other disorder of cranium, neck, eyes, ears, nose, sinuses, teeth, mouth, or other facial or cervical structure.

12. Headache attributed to psychiatric disorder.
- 12.1. Headache attributed to somatization disorder.
- 12.1. Headache attributed to psychotic disorder.

Table 3.3 Painful lesions of the cranial nerves, other facial pain, and other headache disorders—Part III of ICHD-3 (groups 13 and 14)

13. Painful lesions of the cranial nerves and other facial pain
13.1. Pain attributed to a lesion or disease of the trigeminal nerve.
13.2. Pain attributed to a lesion or disease of the glossopharyngeal nerve.
13.3. Pain attributed to a lesion or disease of nervus intermedius.
13.4. Occipital neuralgia
13.5. Neck-tongue syndrome.
13.6. Painful optic neuritis.
13.7. Headache attributed to ischaemic ocular motor nerve palsy.
13.8. Tolosa-hunt syndrome.
13.9. Paratrigeminal oculosympathetic (Raeder's) syndrome.
13.10. Recurrent painful ophthalmoplegic neuropathy.
13.11. Burning mouth syndrome.
13.12. Persistent idiopathic facial pain.
13.13. Central neuropathic pain.
14 Other headache disorders.
14.1. Headache not elsewhere classified.
14.2. Headache unspecified.

References

1. Magiorkinis E, Diamantis A, Mitsikostas DD. Headaches in antiquity and during the early scientific era. J Neurol. 2009;256(8):1215–20.
2. Karenberg A, Leitz C. Headache in magical and medical papyri of ancient Egypt. Cephalalgia. 2001;21(9):911–6.
3. Wolff HG. Headache mechanisms. Mcgill Med J. 1946;15:127–69.
4. Silva-Néto R. Cefaleia: aspectos históricos e tópicos relevantes. Teresina: Halley; 2013.
5. Robertson S, Goodell H, Wolff HG. Headache: the teeth as a source of headache and other pain. Arch Neurol Psychiatr. 1947;57(3):277–91.
6. Kunkle EC, Ray BS, Wolff HG. Studies on headache: the mechanisms and significance of the headache associated with brain tumor. Bull N Y Acad Med. 1942;18(6):400–22.
7. Silva-Néto RP. The study of headache in the 1950s in Latin America by Edgard Raffaelli Júnior (1930-2006). Headache. 2015;55(5):713–7.
8. Silva-Néto RP. Quem foi Edgard Raffaelli Jr. Migrâneas Cefaleias. 2006;9(4):152–8.
9. Ad Hoc Headache Classification Committee. Classification of headache. JAMA. 1962;179(3):717–8.
10. Headache Classification Subcommittee of the International Headache Society. The international classification of headache disorders. Cephalalgia. 1988;8(7):10–96.
11. Headache Classification Subcommittee of the International Headache Society. The international classification of headache disorders, 2nd edition. Cephalalgia. 2004;24(1):8–160.
12. Headache classification Subcommittee of the International Headache Society. The international classification of headache disorders, 3rd edition (beta version). Cephalalgia. 2013;33(9):629–808.
13. Headache Classification Subcommittee of the International Headache Society. The international classification of headache disorders, 3rd edition. Cephalalgia. 2018;38(1):1–211.

Chapter 4
Epidemiology

Epidemiology has saved more lives than all therapeutics

Hector Abad Gómez (1921–1987)

Prevalence

Hypnic headache is considered a rare headache or has very low prevalence in all case series or reviews that have been published, possibly because it is underdiagnosed, as many physicians are unaware of it [1]. Despite this, the statement that it is rare does not reflect its prevalence. According to the cultured norm, rare is that which is not common, abundant, or frequent.

In search of quantitative data, a recent study classified all headaches of the International Classification of Headache Disorders, second Edition (ICHD-2) [2], as for lifetime prevalence, in four classes: very common (>10%), frequent (between 1% and 10%), occasional (between 0.07% and 1%), and rare (<0.07%). In this classification, hypnic headache was categorized as occasional [3].

Since the first description of hypnic headache in 1988 [4], several cases have been reported successively, but little research has shown its true prevalence. Until 1996, only 8 cases had been described [5], but, in 1997, at the eighth International Headache Congress, in Amsterdam (Germany), 36 new cases were presented [6]. In 2003, the first four cases were published in Germany, which represented approximately 0.1% of all headache patients seen at a headache clinic over a 4-year period [7].

A total of 1131 headache patients, of which 239 (21.1%) were aged 60 years or over were studied at a headache center in Brazil. Hypnic headache was diagnosed in only one patient in the elderly sample. Considering all patients, elderly and young, hypnic headache corresponded to 0.09% of patients with headache [8].

In Italy, a study similar to the Brazilian study was carried out from 1998 to 2002 and found this same prevalence of 0.09% in all patients treated with headache [9].

R. Silva-Néto, D. Holle-Lee, *Hypnic Headache*,
https://doi.org/10.1007/978-3-031-32263-1_4

From these findings, some authors stated that the prevalence of hypnic headache is less than 1% of all primary headaches [10].

In 2008, a study was carried out in Greece with 72 patients with headache during sleep. A single case was found that met all diagnostic criteria for hypnic headache, corresponding to 1.4% of the total sample [11]. During the period 1998 to 2006, a Taiwanese study evaluated 1106 headache patients, of which 17 complained of frequent sleep-related headaches and were diagnosed with hypnic headache, showing a prevalence of 0.28% [12].

So far, 11 large case series (≥10 patients per series) of hypnic headache have been published in adult patients [12–22], which corresponded to 65% (223/343) of all cases already published [23]. In just four of them, the prevalence of hypnic headache was determined [12, 16, 18, 22].

A prevalence of 0.07% was estimated in the first case series. Perhaps it was inaccurate as it was based on the diagnosis of hypnic headache for each 1400 headache patients evaluated in a tertiary service [22]. In the second case series, a description of 17 patients represented 0.28% of all patients seen at a headache clinic [12]. The third case series showed a prevalence of 1.1%, diagnosing 13 patients with hypnic headache in a sample of 1180 patients with headache [18]. Finally, in a sample of 11,360 headache patients, 25 cases of hypnic headache were diagnosed, resulting in a prevalence of 0.22% [16].

In 2019, a review of 348 cases of hypnic headache (343 adults and 5 children), from 1988 to 2018, was carried out [23]. This number of cases refers only to those published in articles indexed in the main databases. For this reason, some cases described, including Brazilians, were not included in this series [24, 25]. In addition to these 348 cases, two more were published in the period from 2019 to 2022 [26, 27].

The prevalence of hypnic headache has always been based on retrospective clinical studies. In 2020, the first population-based prevalence study on hypnic headache was conducted in Iceland. In this study, 1398 adults were asked to answer a questionnaire with several questions about headache. One of the questions was about hypnic headache: “Do you have a headache that occurs only during sleep and causes wakening?” A neurologist interviewed those who answered “YES” to this question to confirm the diagnosis of hypnic headache based on ICHD-3β [28].

Only 921 (519 women and 402 men) adults participated in the study, with a mean age of 45.6 ± 13.2 years. A total of six participants (0.7%), all women, answered “YES” to the hypnic headache screening question. After an interview with a neurologist, only two women had probable hypnic headache, resulting in a prevalence of 0.22%. None had definitive hypnic headache [28].

This book addressed the clinical characteristics, pathophysiology, and treatment of hypnic headache, as detailed in Tables 4.1 and 4.2. It was based on the largest series of cases [12–22] and found that the prevalence of hypnic headache in adults ranged from 0.07 to 0.28% [8, 9, 12, 16, 22].

Hypnic headache is not exclusive to adults as established in the initial criteria for this headache disorder. There is a predominance after the age of 50 years, but children also have hypnic headache. In the review of 348 cases of hypnic headache,

Table 4.1 Distribution of the 345 adults with hypnic headache from 1988 to 2022, according to age and sex

Author (s), Year	Number of cases	Age or average age (years)	Sex	
			Male	Female
Raskin, 1988 [4]	6	71.3	5	1
Newman et al., 1990 [29]	2	75	–	2
Goadsby and Lipton, 1997 [30]	1	84	–	1
Gould et al., 1997 [31]	1	65	–	1
Queiroz and Coral, 1997 [32]	1	59	1	–
Skobieranda et al., 1997 [33]	6	60–78	NR	NR
Dodick et al., 1998 [22]	19	60.5	3	16
Ivañez et al., 1998 [5]	1	74	1	–
Morales-Asín et al., 1998 [6]	3	75.3	1	2
Klimek and Sklodowski, 1999 [34]	2	50.5	2	–
Pérez-Martínez et al., 1999 [35]	1	70	–	1
Arjona et al., 2000 [36]	1	79	–	1
Dodick et al., 2000 [37]	3	57.7	2	1
Trucco et al., 2000 [38]	1	83	1	–
Zanchin et al., 2000 [39]	1	72	–	1
Centonze et al., 2001 [40]	1	47	1	–
Martins and Gouveia, 2001 [41]	1	68	–	1
Capo and Esposito, 2001 [42]	1	72	1	–
Vieira Dias and Esperança, 2002 [43]	4	57.0	1	3
Ghiotto et al., 2002 [44]	8	64.5	4	4
Pinto et al., 2002 [45]	8	58.5	1	7
Relja et al., 2002 [46]	2	74.0	1	1
Brooks et al., 2003 [47]	1	67	–	1
Evers et al., 2003 [7]	4	64.5	1	3
Pinessi et al., 2003 [48]	2	53.5	1	1
Sibon et al., 2003 [49]	1	68	–	1
Kocasoy Orhan et al., 2004 [50]	1	NR	–	1
Lisotto et al., 2004 [9]	4	71.2	1	3
Manni et al., 2004 [21]	10	67.9	4	6
Patsouros et al., 2004 [51]	1	60	–	1
Buzzi et al., 2005 [52]	1	70	–	1
Capuano et al., 2005 [53]	1	54	–	1
Domitrz, 2005 [54]	2	55.0	1	1
Dolso et al., 2006 [55]	1	40	1	–
Evans, 2006 [56]	1	56	–	1
Fukuhara et al., 2006 [57]	3	61.3	–	3
Guido and Specchio, 2006 [58]	1	67	–	1
Kerr et al., 2006 [59]	1	79	1	–
Peters et al., 2006 [60]	1	58	1	–

(continued)

Table 4.1 (continued)

Author (s), Year	Number of cases	Age or average age (years)	Sex	
			Male	Female
Porta-Etessam et al., 2006 [61]	8	NR	4	4
Schürks et al., 2006 [62]	1	71	–	1
Ulrich, 2006 [63]	1	78	–	1
Garza and Swanson, 2007 [64]	1	53	1	–
Marziniak et al., 2007 [65]	1	58	–	1
Antunno et al., 2008 [66]	1	63	–	1
Liang et al., 2008 [12]	17	69.6	9	8
Mitsikostas et al., 2008 [11]	1	68	–	1
Prakash and Dahbi, 2008 [67]	1	19	1	–
Seidel et al., 2008 [68]	1	54	–	1
Donnet and Lantéri-Minet, 2009 [20]	22	60.5	10	12
Porta-Etessam et al., 2009 [69]	1	36	1	–
Karlovasitou et al., 2009 [70]	1	54	–	1
Caminero et al., 2010 [71]	2	61.0	1	1
Holle et al., 2010 [19]	20	67.5	7	13
Bender, 2012 [72]	1	45	–	1
Dolezil and Mavrokordatos, 2012 [73]	1	64	–	1
Jiménez-Caballero et al., 2012 [17]	24	63–68	9	15
Mulero et al., 2012 [18]	13	56.7	2	11
Ouahmane et al., 2012 [74]	2	60,0	1	1
Son et al., 2012 [75]	1	64	–	1
Peng et al., 2013 [76]	2	55.5	1	1
Porta-Etessam et al., 2013 [77]	6	60.7	3	3
Silva-Néto and Almeida, 2014 [16]	25	72.5	5	20
Ruiz et al., 2015 [14]	23	56.2	4	19
Escudero Martínez et al., 2015 [15]	10	52.1	1	9
Arai, 2015 [78]	1	81	–	1
Aguirre-Rodríguez et al., 2016 [79]	1	46	NR	NR
Tariq et al., 2016 [13]	40	62.0	8	32
Fantini et al., 2016 [80]	1	49	–	1
Rehmann et al., 2017 [81]	1	74	–	1
Dissanayake et al., 2017 [82]	1	86	–	1
Pérez Hernández and Ontañón, 2017 [83]	1	41	–	1
Zhang et al., 2019 [26]	1	58	1	–
Kesserwani, 2021 [27]	1	48	–	1

NR: Not reported
Source: Silva-Néto RP, Sousa-Santos PEM, Peres MFP. Hypnic headache: A review of 348 cases published from 1988 to 2018. J Neurol Sci 2019;401:103–9

Table 4.2 Distribution of the five children with hypnic headache from 1988 to 2022, according age and sex

Author (s), Year	Number of cases	Age or average age (years)	Sex	
			Male	Female
Cerminara et al., 2011 [84]	3	9.3	2	1
Scagni and Pagliero, 2008 [85]	1	8	–	1
Grosberg et al., 2004 [86]	1	9	–	1

Source: Silva-Néto RP, Almeida KJ. Hypnic headache in childhood: A literature review. J Neurol Sci 2015;356 [1, 2]:45–8

five cases in the pediatric age group were described [84–86]. See more details in Chap. 5.

The 350 cases of hypnic headache described in the period from 1988 to 2022 [23, 26, 27, 87] were all classified, according to ICHD-3 [1], as primary or idiopathic headache, that is, their cause was not attributed to another pathology. Another 16 cases were due to other diseases, featuring a secondary hypnic headache [88–103], as shown in Table 4.3.

According to ICHD-3, hypnic headache has well-defined diagnostic criteria and is not attributed to another disorder [104]. However, there are other headaches that also occur during sleep or when waking up, but are secondary to other pathologies. Therefore, it is necessary to make a differential diagnosis with all forms of headache that have a nocturnal rhythm. Obviously, the clinical history is fundamental for this diagnosis and the investigation with complementary exams must be evaluated according to the evidence of the case.

Of the 16 patients with secondary hypnic headache, there were 6 men and 10 women. The mean age of patients was 59.9 ± 15.0 years, ranging from 20 to 84 years. The causes of hypnic headache were attributed to cranial vascular disorder (five), to non-vascular intracranial disorder (six), to a substance or its withdrawal (two), and to disorder of homeostasis (three), as shown in Table 4.3.

Table 4.3 Distribution of 16 cases of secondary hypnic headache published from 1988 to 2022, according to age, sex, and etiology

Etiology	Author (s), Year	Cases	Age (year)	Sex (M/F)
Attributed to cranial vascular disorder				
Pontine ischemic injury	Moon et al., 2006 [88]	1	71	M
Idiopathic cyclic edema	Godoy, 2010 [89]	1	56	M
Basilar artery dolichoectasia	Moreira et al., 2015 [90]	1	69	F
Basilar artery dolichoectasia	Fonseca et al., 2016 [91]	1	54	M
Intracranial aneurysm	Alfred et al., 2022 [92]	1	20	F
Attributed to non-vascular intracranial disorder				
Posterior fossa meningioma	Peatfield et al., 2003 [93]	1	54	F
Nonfunctioning pituitary macroadenoma	Garza et al., 2009 [94]	1	74	F
GH-secreting pituitary tumor	Valentinis et al. 2009 [95]	1	66	M
Hemangioblastoma of the cerebellum	Mullally et al., 2010 [96]	1	58	M
Acoustic neuroma	Ceronie et al., 2021 [97]	1	40	F
Intracranial hypotension	Freeman et al., 2004 [98]	1	80	M
Attributed to a substance or its withdrawal				
Medication-overuse headache	Baykan et al., 2008 [99]	1	54	F
ACE inhibitor withdrawal	Eccles et al., 2007 [100]	1	84	F
Attributed to disorder of homeostasis				
Nocturnal arterial hypertension	Silva-Néto et al., 2013 [101]	1	60	F
Nocturnal arterial hypertension	Gil-Gouveia et al., 2007 [102]	1	54	F
Nocturnal hypoglycemia	Silva-Néto et al., 2019 [103]	1	64	F

F: female; M: male; ACE: angiotensin converting enzyme; GH: growing hormone.
Source: Fortes YML, Erudilho E, Silva TS, Souza WPO, Silva-Néto RP. Secondary hypnic headache: A literature review in the last 34 years. Headache Medicine 2022;13 [3]:163–6

Geographic Distribution

Many diseases can be influenced by the physical and phenotypic characteristics (race) of an individual or predominate in a group of people who share the same geographical or social origin (ethnicity), such as sickle cell anemia, high blood pressure, and diabetes mellitus.

In the case of hypnic headache, it seems that this influence does not exist. In the analysis of the geographical distribution of the 350 published idiopathic cases, it is noted that this rare disorder is a disease without borders. It occurs on all continents (Fig. 4.1) and, probably, the predominance of publications in some countries is only due to the advance in the study of headache. Currently, Spain is the country with the highest number of cases of hypnic headache (99 cases), the USA is the second (81

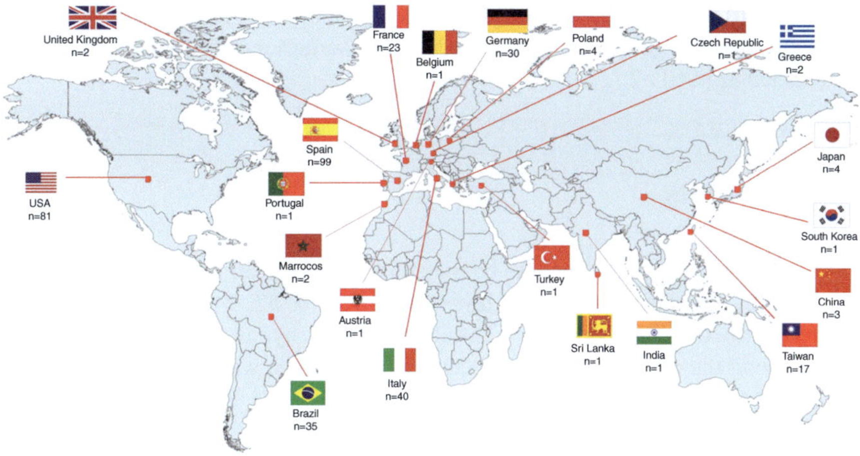

Fig. 4.1 Geographical distribution of 350 cases of hypnic headache published from 1988 to 2022

cases), Italy is the third (40 cases), Brazil is the fourth (35 cases), and Germany is the fifth (30 cases) [23, 87].

Sex

In the first six hypnic headache patients described by Raskin, in 1988, there was a predominance of males, with five men and one woman (all were adults) [4]. From the publications of the large case series, a female prevalence began to be observed. To date, 345 cases of hypnic headache have been described in adult patients, in which gender was reported in 338 of them. The predominance was female (68.6% versus 31.4%) (Table 4.1). The female/male ratio was 2.2:1 [23, 87].

Age of Onset of Pain

According to the current diagnostic criteria for hypnic headache, the onset of headache attacks can occur at any age [104], but in the past, this criterion established the onset of pain after 50 years of age [2]. Raskin, initially made this statement in 1998, when describing six patients with a mean age of onset of pain of 71.3 ± 4.5 years [4].

In the most recent review of 345 adult patients with hypnic headache, the age of onset of pain was 58.0 ± 13.1 years, ranging from 15 to 85 years. In only 9% of them, the pain started below the age of 50 years. It was based on the chronological age at which the patient was treated and the time of pain until diagnosis, in order to know the age of onset of pain [23, 26, 27]. From these data, it was understood that pain does not occur, for the first time, exclusively after the age of 50 years. Therefore, the age of onset of pain should not be a diagnostic criterion for hypnic headache, as established in ICHD-2 [2].

Family History

Hypnic headache does not seem to be transmitted from generation to generation, as this hereditary character has been investigated [7, 50, 52, 54, 65, 67, 78]. In the cases described, no patient with a family history of hypnic headache was found [23]. Among the other primary headaches, only migraine was mentioned in family relationships, such as mother, children, or grandchildren [5, 20, 30].

References

1. Holle D, Naegel S, Obermann M. Hypnic headache. Cephalalgia. 2013;33(16):1349–57.
2. Headache Classification Subcommittee of the International Headache Society. The international classification of headache disorders, 2nd edition. Cephalalgia. 2004;24(1):8–160.
3. Valença MM, Oliveira DA. The frequent unusual headache syndromes: a proposed classification based on lifetime prevalence. Headache. 2016;56(1):141–52.
4. Raskin NH. The hypnic headache syndrome. Headache. 1988;28(8):534–6.
5. Ivañez V, Soler R, Barreiro P. Hypnic headache syndrome: a case with good response to indomethacin. Cephalalgia. 1998;18(4):225–6.
6. Morales-Asín F, Mauri JA, Iñiguez C, Espada F, Mostacero E. The hypnic headache syndrome: report of three new cases. Cephalalgia. 1998;18(3):157–8.
7. Evers S, Rahmann A, Schwaag S, Lüdermann P, Husstedt IW. Hypnic headache – the first German cases including polysomnography. Cephalalgia. 2003;23(1):20–3.
8. Souza JA, Moreira Filho PF, Jevoux CC, Albertino S, Sarmento EM, Brito CM. Idade como um fator de risco independente para cefaleias secundárias. Arq Neuropsiquiatr. 2004;62(4):1038–45.
9. Lisoto C, Mainardi F, Maggioni F, Zanchin G. Episodic hypnic headache? Cephalalgia. 2004;24(8):681–5.
10. Casucci G, d'Onofrio F, Torelli P. Rare primary headaches: clinical insights. Neurol Sci. 2004;25(3):77–83.
11. Mitsikostas DD, Vikelis M, Viskos A. Refractory chronic headache associated with obstructive sleep apnoea syndrome. Cephalalgia. 2008;28(2):139–43.
12. Liang JF, Fuh JL, Yu HY, Hsu CY, Wang SJ. Clinical features, polysomnography and outcome in patients with hypnic headache. Cephalalgia. 2008;28(3):209–15.
13. Tariq N, Estemalik E, Vij B, Kriegler JS, Tepper SJ, Stillman MJ. Long-term outcomes and clinical characteristics of hypnic headache syndrome: 40 patients series from a tertiary referral center. Headache. 2016;56(4):717–24.
14. Ruiz M, Mulero P, Pedraza MI, de la Cruz C, Rodríguez C, Muñoz I, et al. From wakefulness to sleep: migraine and hypnic headache association in a series of 23 patients. Headache. 2015;55(1):167–73.
15. Escudero Martínez I, González-Oria C, Bernal Sánchez-Arjona M, Jiménez Hernández MD. Description of series of 10 patients with hypnic headache: discussion of the diagnostic criteria. Neurologia. 2015;30(4):195–200.

16. Silva-Néto RP, Almeida KJ. Hypnic headache: a descriptive study of 25 new cases in Brazil. J Neurol Sci. 2014;338(1–2):166–8.
17. Jiménez-Caballero PE, Gámez-Leyva G, Gómez M, Casado-Naranjo I. Descripción de una serie de casos de cefalea hípnica. Diferenciación entre sexos Rev Neurol. 2012;54(6):332–6.
18. Mulero P, Guerrero-Peral AL, Cortijo E, Jabary NS, Herrero-Velázquez S, Miranda S, et al. Cefalea hípnica: características de una serie de 13 nuevos casos y propuesta de modificación de los criterios diagnósticos. Rev Neurol. 2012;54(3):129–36.
19. Holle D, Naegel S, Krebs S, Katsarava Z, Diener HC, Gaul C, et al. Clinical characteristics and therapeutic options in hypnic headache. Cephalalgia. 2010;30(12):1435–42.
20. Donnet A, Lantéri-Minet M. A consecutive series of 22 cases of hypnic headache in France. Cephalalgia. 2009;29(9):928–34.
21. Manni R, Sances G, Terzaghi M, Ghiotto N, Nappi G. Hypnic headache: PSG evidence of both REM-and NREM-related attacks. Neurology. 2004;62(8):1411–3.
22. Dodick DW, Mosek AC, Campbell JK. The hypnic ('alarm clock') headache syndrome. Cephalalgia. 1998;18(3):152–6.
23. Silva-Néto RP, Sousa-Santos PEM, Peres MFP. Hypnic headache: a review of 348 cases published from 1988 to 2018. J Neurol Sci. 2019;401:103–9.
24. Almeida RF, Leão IMT, Gomes JBL. Cefaleia hípnica. Migrâneas e Cefaleias. 2007;10(1):20–3.
25. Marrone LCP, Trentin S, Oliveira FM, Marrone ACH. Cefaléia hípnica em adulto jovem – relato de caso. Rev Bras Neurol. 2010;46(1):31–3.
26. Zhang Y, Wang C, Chen Y, Wang R, Lian Y. Hypnic headache with dopaminergic neuron dysfunction: new insight from a rare case. Pain Med. 2019;20(8):1639–42.
27. Kesserwani H. Hypnic headache responds to topiramate: a case report and a review of mechanisms of action of therapeutic agents. Cureus. 2021;13(3):e13790.
28. Eliasson JH, Scher AI, Buse DC, Tietjen G, Lipton RB, Launer LJ, et al. The prevalence of hypnic headache in Iceland. Cephalalgia. 2020;40(8):863–5.
29. Newman LC, Lipton RB, Solomon S. The hypnic headache syndrome: a benign headache disorder of the elderly. Neurology. 1990;40(12):1904–5.
30. Goadsby PJ, Lipton RB. A review of paroxysmal hemicranias, SUNCT syndrome and other short-lasting headaches with autonomic feature, including new cases. Brain. 1997;120(1):193–209.
31. Gould JD, Silberstein SD. Unilateral hypnic headache: a case study. Neurology. 1997;49(6):1749–51.
32. Queiroz LP, Coral LC. The hypnic headache syndrome – a case report (Abstract). Proceedings of 8th Congress of the International Headache Society, 1997 Jun 10–14; Amsterdam, Germany. Cephalalgia. 1997;17(3):303.
33. Skobieranda FG, Lee TG, Solomon GD. The hypnic headache syndrome: six additional patients (Abstract). Proceedings of 8th congress of the international headache society, 1997 Jun 10-14; Amsterdam, Germany. Cephalalgia. 1997;17(3):304–5.
34. Klimek A, Sklodowski P, Night headache. Report of 2 cases. Neurol Neurochir Pol. 1999;33(5):49–54.
35. Perez-Martinez DA, Berbel-Garcia A, Puente-Muñoz AI, Saiz-Diaz RA, de Toledo-Heras M, Porta-Etessam J, et al. Hypnic headache: a new case. Rev Neurol. 1999;28(9):883–4.
36. Arjona JA, Jimenez-Jimenez FJ, Vela-Bueno A, Tallon-Barranco A. Hypnic headache associated with stage 3 slow wave sleep. Headache. 2000;40(9):753–4.
37. Dodick DW, Jones JM, Capobianco DJ. Hypnic headache: another indomethacin-responsive headache syndrome? Headache. 2000;40(10):830–5.
38. Trucco M, Maggioni F, Badino R, Zanchin G. Hypnic headache syndrome: report of a new Italian case. Cephalalgia. 2000;20(4):312.
39. Zanchin G, Lisotto C, Maggioni F. The hypnic headache syndrome: the first description of an Italian case. J Headache Pain. 2000;1(1):60.

40. Centonze V, D'Amico D, Usai S, Causarano V, Bassi A, Bussone G. First Italian case of hypnic headache, with literature review and discussion of nosology. Cephalalgia. 2001;21(1):71–4.
41. Martins IP, Gouveia RG. Hypnic headache and travel across time zones: a case report. Cephalalgia. 2001;21(9):928–31.
42. Capo G, Esposito A. Hypnic headache. A new Italian case with a good response to pizotifene and melatonin (Abstract). Proceedings of 10th congress of the international headache society, 2001 Jun 29 to Jul 3; New York, EUA. Cephalalgia. 2001;21(4):505–6.
43. Vieira-Dias M, Esperança P. Hypnic headache: a report of four cases. Rev Neurol. 2002;34(10):950–1.
44. Ghiotto N, Sances G, Di Lorenzo G, Trucco M, Loi M, Sandrini G, et al. Report of eight new cases of hypnic headache and mini-review of the literature. Funct Neurol. 2002;17(4):211–9.
45. Pinto CAR, Fragoso YD, Souza Carvalho D, Gabbai AA. Hypnic headache syndrome: clinical aspects of eight patients in Brazil. Cephalalgia. 2002;22(10):824–7.
46. Relja G, Zorzon M, Locatelli L, Carraro N, Antonello RM, Cazzato G. Hypnic headache: rapid and long-lasting response to prednisone in two new cases. Cephalalgia. 2002;22(2):157–9.
47. Brooks PT, Hadjikoutis S, Pickersgill TP. Lithium responsive hypnic headache in a patient with multiple sclerosis (Abstract). Proceedings of Association of British Neurologists Spring Meeting, 2003 Apr 2–4; Cardiff, UK. J Neurol Neurosurg Psychiatry. 2003;74(10):1459.
48. Pinessi L, Rainero I, Cicolin A, Zibetti M, Gentile S, Mutani R. Hypnic headache syndrome: association of the attacks with REM sleep. Cephalalgia. 2003;23(2):150–4.
49. Sibon I, Ghorayeb I, Henry P. Successful treatment of hypnic headache syndrome with acetazolamide. Neurology. 2003;61(8):1157–8.
50. Kocasoy-Orhan E, Kayrak-Ertas N, Orhan KS, Ertas M. Hypnic headache syndrome: excessive periodic limb movements in polysomnography. Agri. 2004;16(4):28–30.
51. Patsouros N, Laloux P, Ossemann M. Hypnic headache: a case report with polysomnography. Acta Neurol Belg. 2004;104(1):37–40.
52. Buzzi MG, Cologno D, Formisano R, Caltagirone C. Hypnic headache responsive to indomethacin: second Italian case. Funct Neurol. 2005;20(2):85–7.
53. Capuano A, Vollono C, Rubino M, Mei D, Cali C, De Angelis A, et al. Hypnic headache: actigraphic and polysomnographic study of a case. Cephalalgia. 2005;25(6):466–9.
54. Domitrz I. Hypnic headache as a primary short-lasting night headache: a report of two cases. Neurol Neurochir Pol. 2005;39(1):77–9.
55. Dolso P, Merlino G, Fratticci L, Canesin R, Valiante G, Coccolo D, et al. Non-REM hypnic headache: a circadian disorder? A clinical and polysomnography Cephalalgia. 2006;27(1):83–6.
56. Evans RW, Dodick DW, Schwedt TJ. The headaches that awaken us. Headache. 2006;46(4):678–81.
57. Fukuhara Y, Takeshima T, Ishizaki K, Burioka N, Nakashima K. Three Japanese cases of hypnic headache. Rinsho Shinkeigaku. 2006;46(2):148–53.
58. Guido M, Specchio LM. Successful treatment of hypnic headache with topiramate: a case report. Headache. 2006;46(7):1205–6.
59. Kerr E, Hewitt R, Gleadhill I. Benign headache in the elderly – a case report of hypnic headache. Ulster Med J. 2006;75(2):158–9.
60. Peters N, Lorenzl S, Fischereder J, Bötzel K, Straube A. Hypnic headache: a case presentation including polysomnography. Cephalalgia. 2006;26(1):84–6.
61. Porta-Etessam J, Pérez-Martínez DA, Martínez-Salio A, Berbel-García A, Gordo R. Successful treatment of hypnic headache syndrome with flunarizine (Abstract). Proceedings of 8th Headache Congress of the European Headache Federation, 2006 Apr 26–29; Valencia, Spain. J Headache Pain. 2006;7(1):56.
62. Schürks M, Kastrup O, Diener HC. Triptan responsive hypnic headache? Eur J Neurol. 2006;13(6):666–72.
63. Ulrich K, Gunreben B, Lang E, Sitti R, Griessinger N. Pregabalin in the therapy of hypnic headache. Cephalalgia. 2006;26(8):1031–2.

64. Garza I, Swanson J. Successful preventive therapy in hypnic headache using hypnotics: a case report. Cephalalgia. 2007;27(9):1080–1.
65. Marziniak M, Voss J, Evers S. Hypnic headache successfully treated with botulinum toxin type a. Cephalalgia. 2007;27(9):1082–4.
66. Autunno M, Messina C, Blandino A, Rodolico C. Hypnic headache responsive to low-dose topiramate: a case report. Headache. 2008;48(2):292–4.
67. Prakash S, Dahbi AS. Relapsing remitting hypnic headache responsive to indomethacin in an adolescent: a case report. J Headache Pain. 2008;9(6):393–5.
68. Seidel S, Zeitlhofer J, Wöber C. First Austrian case of hypnic headache: serial polysomnography and blood pressure monitoring in treatment with indomethacin. Cephalalgia. 2008;28(10):1086–90.
69. Porta-Etessam JP, García-Morales I, Di Capua D, García-Cobos R. A patient with primary sexual headache associated with hypnic headaches. J Headache Pain. 2009;10(2):135.
70. Karlovasitou A, Avdelidi E, Andriopoulou G, Baloyannis S. Transient hypnic headache syndrome in a patient with bipolar disorder after the withdrawal of long-term lithium treatment: a case report. Cephalalgia. 2009;29(4):484–6.
71. Caminero AB, Martín J, Del Río MS. Secondary hypnic headache or symptomatic nocturnal hipertensión? Two case reports Cephalalgia. 2010;30(9):1137–9.
72. Bender SD. An unusual case of hypnic headache ameliorated utilizing a mandibular advancement oral appliance. Sleep Breath. 2012;16(3):599–602.
73. Dolezil D, Mavrokordatos C. Hypnic headache- a rare primary headache disorder with very good response to indomethacin. Neuro Endocrinol Lett. 2012;33(6):597–9.
74. Ouahmane Y, Mounach J, Satte A, Zerhouni A, Ouhabi H. Hypnic headache: response to lamotrigine in two cases. Cephalalgia. 2012;32(8):645–8.
75. Son BC, Yang SH, Hong JT, Lee SW. Occipital nerve stimulation for medically refractory hypnic headache. Neuromodulation. 2012;15(4):381–6.
76. Peng H, Wang L, He B, Giudice M, Zhang L, Zhao ZX. Hypnic headache responsive to sodium ferulate in 2 new cases. Clin J Pain. 2013;29(1):89–91.
77. Porta-Etessam J, Muñiz S, Cuadrado ML, González-García N, Orviz A, Abarrategui B, et al. Successful treatment of hypnic headache syndrome with flunarizine. J Neurol Neurosci. 2013;(4)1:2.
78. Arai M. A case of unilateral hypnic headache: rapid response to ramelteon, a selective melatonin MT1/MT2 receptor agonist. Headache. 2015;55(7):1010–1.
79. Aguirre-Rodríguez CJ, Hernández-Martínez N, Aguirre-Rodríguez FJ. Cefalea hípnica, a propósito de un caso. SEMERGEN. 2016;42(2):12–3.
80. Fantini J, Granato A, Zorzon M, Manganotti P. Case report: coexistence of SUNCT and hypnic headache in the same patient. Headache. 2016;56(9):1503–6.
81. Rehmann R, Tegenthoff M, Zimmer C, Stude P. Case report of an alleviation of pain symptoms in hypnic headache via greater occipital nerve block. Cephalalgia. 2017;37(10):998–1000.
82. Dissanayake KP, Wanniarachchi DP, Ranawaka UK. Case report of hypnic headache: a rare headache disorder with nocturnal symptoms. BMC Res Notes. 2017;10(1):318.
83. Pérez Hernández A, Gómez OE. Influenza a virus: a possible trigger factor for hypnic headache? Neurologia. 2017;32(1):67–8.
84. Cerminara C, Compagnone E, Coniglio A, Margiotta M, Curatolo P, Villa MP, et al. Hypnic headache in children. Cephalalgia. 2011;31(16):1673–6.
85. Scagni P, Pagliero R. Hypnic in childhood: a new report. J Paediatr Child Health. 2008;44(1–2):83–4.
86. Grosberg BM, Lipton RB, Solomon S, Ballaban-Gil K. Hypnic headache in childhood? A case report Cephalalgia. 2004;25(1):68–70.
87. Silva-Néto. Cefaleia hípnica: Dores que vem pelo sono. Nova Aliança: Teresina; 2019.
88. Moon HS, Chung CS, Hong SB, Kim YB, Chung PW. A case of symptomatic hypnic headache syndrome. Cephalalgia. 2006;26(1):81–3.

89. Godoy JM. Remission of hypnic headache associated with idiopathic cyclic edema with the use of aminaphtone. Open Neurol J. 2010;4:90–1.
90. Moreira IM, Mendonça T, Monteiro JP, Santos E. Hypnic headache and basilar artery dolichoectasia. Neurologist. 2015;20(6):106–7.
91. Fonseca M, Teotónio P, Fonseca AC. An unsuspected cause of hypnic-like headache. J Neurol. 2016;264(2):404–6.
92. Aldred MP, Raviskanthan S, Mortensen PW, Lee AG. Hypnic headaches in a patient post coiling and clipping of intracranial aneurysm. J Neuroophthalmol. 2021;42(1):415–6.
93. Peatfield RC, Mendoza ND. Posterior fossa meningioma presenting as hypnic headache. Headache. 2003;43(9):1007–8.
94. Garza I, Oas KH. Symptomatic hypnic headache secondary to a nonfunctioning pituitary macroadenoma. Headache. 2009;49(3):470–2.
95. Valentinis L, Tuniz F, Mucchiut M, Vindigni M, Skrap M, Bergonzi P, et al. Hypnic headache secondary to a growth hormone-secreting pituitary tumour. Cephalalgia. 2008;29(1):82–4.
96. Mullally WJ, Hall KE. Hypnic headache secondary to haemangioblastoma of the cerebellum. Cephalalgia. 2010;30(7):887–9.
97. Ceronie B, Green F, Cockerell OC. Acoustic neuroma presenting as a hypnic headache. BMJ Case Rep. 2021;14(3):e235830.
98. Freeman WD, Brazis TW, Capobianco DJ, Lamer T. Hypnic headache and intracranial hypotension. In: Proceedings of 46th Annual Scientific Meeting American Headache Society, 2004 Jun 10–13; Vancouver, British Columbia. Headache. 2004;44(5):498.
99. Baykan B, Ertas M. Hypnic headache associated with medication overuse: case report. Agri. 2008;20(3):40–3.
100. Eccles MJ, Gutowski NJ. Precipitation of long duration hypnic headaches after ACE inhibitor withdrawal. J Neurol. 2007;254(11):1597–8.
101. Silva-Néto RP, Bernardino SN. Ambulatory blood pressure monitoring in patient with hypnic headache: a case study. Headache. 2013;53(7):1157–8.
102. Gil-Gouveia R, Goadsby PJ. Secondary hypnic headache. J Neurol. 2007;254(5):646–54.
103. Silva-Néto RP, Soares AA, Peres MFP. Hypnic headache due to hypoglycemia: a case report. Headache. 2019;59(8):1370–3.
104. Headache Classification Subcommittee of the International Headache Society. The international classification of headache disorders, 3rd edition. Cephalalgia. 2018;38(1):1–211.

Chapter 5
Clinical Characteristics in Adults

Medicine has made steady progress for a century, inventing thousands of new diseases

Louis Scutenaire (1905–1987)

Introduction

Semiological characteristics of pain, such as onset, time, location, character, intensity, frequency, duration, and associated symptoms are not part of the diagnostic criteria for hypnic headache. These characteristics are not considered in the current diagnostic criteria for hypnic headache [1], as shown in Table 5.1, but they are extremely important in the diagnostic accuracy.

Diagnosis of hypnic headache is eminently clinical, so it is necessary to have a deeper knowledge about its semiology, since the complementary exams do not show any abnormalities, being useful for the differential diagnosis.

Hypnic headache is unknown to many neurologists because its occurrence is rare. If there is a need to establish this diagnosis, the literature should be consulted to know some nuances that are not explicit in the classification of headache.

In this chapter, the clinical and epidemiological characteristics of hypnic headache in adult patients will be studied. They are based on the reports of 345 cases described [2–4] in 76 articles and are summarized in Table 5.2.

Table 5.1 Diagnostics criteria for hypnic headache according to ICHD-3 (2018)

A. Recurrent headache attacks fulfilling criteria B–E.
B. Developing only during sleep and causing wakening.
C. Occurring on ≥10 days/month for >3 months.
D. Lasting from 15 mins up to 4 h after waking.
E. No cranial autonomic symptoms or restlessness.
F. Not better accounted for by another ICHD-3 diagnosis.

R. Silva-Néto, D. Holle-Lee, *Hypnic Headache*,
https://doi.org/10.1007/978-3-031-32263-1_5

Table 5.2 Clinical and Epidemiological Characteristics of the 345 Adult Patients with Hypnic headache

Characteristics	
FEMALE/MALE (%)	68.6/31.4
Age of onset of pain (years)	58.0 ± 13.1 (15–85)
Latency until diagnosis (years)	7.6 ± 14.2 (0.1–39)
Timing of attacks • Daytime naps • 0:00–2:00 a.m. • 2:00–4:00 a.m. • 4:00–6:00 a.m.	5.2 27.6 51.1 16.1
Duration of attacks (minutes) • < 30 • 30–120 • > 120	93.6 ± 65.3 (10–600) 3.4 78.0 18.6
Number of attacks per 24 h • One • Two • ≥ three	1.3 ± 0.6 (1–6) 64.5 29.7 5.8
Frequency (days/month) • < 10 • ≥ 10	21.9 ± 7.6 (3–31) 5.5 94.5
Quality of pain • Dull/pressure • Throbbing/pulsatile • Stabbing/burning	74.4 18.3 7.3
Intensity of pain • Mild (VAS 1–4) • Moderate (VAS 5–7) • Severe (VAS 8–9) • Very severe (VAS 10)	5.5 61.5 32.5 0.8
Localization of pain • Unilateral (57.8% on the left and 42.2% on the right) • Bilateral • Holocranianal/diffuse	30.3 55.5 14.2
Concomitant symptoms • None • Nausea or vomiting (95.8% only nausea) • Photophobia or phonophobia • Photophobia and phonophobia	62.6 21.9 11.9 3.6
Trigemino-autonomics features • Absent • Present (61.1% tearing and 16.7% rhinorrhoea)	92.4 7.6

Note: Data are presented in percentages (%) and/or arithmetic mean ± standard deviation (interval in parentheses). Data were not available from all patients for every aspect; VAS: visual analogue scale

Source: Silva-Néto RP, Sousa-Santos PEM, Peres MFP. Hypnic headache: A review of 348 cases published from 1988 to 2018. J Neurol Sci 2019;401:103–9

Pretreatment Pain Time (Latency)

Unfortunately, from the onset of pain to finding a headache specialist, hypnic headache patients take a few years to be properly diagnosed. This shows that this disorder is few recognized and, perhaps, underdiagnosed. Some studies have shown that this latency time was, on average, 3–8 years [2, 5–8].

In 2005, a review of 94 cases showed that the headache time until diagnosis ranged from 1 to 35 years, with an average of 5 years [6]. In a review of 345 cases, the diagnosis was made, on average, 7 years and 7 months (ranging from 1 month to 39 years) after the onset of headache [2–4].

Time of Onset of Pain

According to ICHD-3, headache develops only during sleep, causing the patient to awaken [1]. Usually, headache attacks occur right after the patient falls asleep and there is often a regular time of pain; hence the name "alarm clock headache." [9, 10]

Awakening by pain does not occur only during night sleep. Some patients present headache during naps or daytime naps [8, 11–17], according to the initial description made by Raskin, in 1988 [18]. In 5.2% of patients, pain occurs during daytime naps [2]. In 0.6% of patients, pain appears during a nightmare [19, 20] and in 3%, during vivid dreams [8, 15–17, 19, 21, 22].

Several studies have found that pain appears at night, after sleep onset, in about 95% of patients [6, 8, 10]. However, approximately one-third of patients are not able to report the exact moment of onset of pain. Therefore, it is essential to use a headache diary for a correct diagnosis of the time of onset of pain, in addition to the frequency and intensity of headache attacks [7].

Nocturnal episodes occur after the patient falls asleep, distributed in the following percentages and times: 27.6%, before 2 o'clock in the morning; 51.1%, between 4 and 4 h; and 16.1%, after 4 hours [2].

Duration of Headache Attacks

Duration of headache attacks has always been a diagnostic criterion for hypnic headache. In the first cases described by Raskin, the pain woke the patients and persisted for 30–60 mins [18]. Headache duration should be 5–60 mins, according to the first diagnostic criteria that have been suggested [23]. A few years later, this duration went from 10 to 180 mins [24].

Finally in ICHD-3, the headache attacks last for more than 15 mins, and can last for up to 4 h after awakening. Also in this classification, in the final comments, it is added that the headache attacks generally last from 15 to 180 mins, but longer durations have been described [1]. In 345 published cases, the headache attacks lasted from 10 to 600 mins, with an average of 90 mins [2–4].

Frequency of Headache Attacks

From the first described cases of hypnic headache, the number of days of headache occurrence was determined. Initially, it was suggested that headache would occur at least 15 times a month for at least 1 month [23, 25].

In the current classification, headache attacks occur on ≥10 days per month, for >3 months. In most cases, the pain is persistent, with daily or almost daily headache, but an episodic subtype (in <15 days/month) can occur [1].

The number of attacks both per 24 h and per month is important. In practice, the number of attacks per 24 h represents events per night. High frequency of headache attacks is a well-known feature of hypnic headache [24, 26, 27]. For this reason, some authors consider two forms of hypnic headache, one chronic and the other episodic, requiring further studies, in the long term, to define the temporal patterns [27]. In Chap. 10, a possible classification of hypnic headache into two forms will be discussed: episodic and chronic.

After analyzing the last 345 published cases of hypnic headache, it was found that, in 94.5% of the patients, headache occurred 10 or more days per month, with an average of 21 days. In 64.5% of patients, only one headache attack occurred at night and at a predictable time during sleep. Two headache attacks occurred in 29.7% and three or more in 5.8% of patients [2–4].

Quality of Pain

Pain quality is not a diagnostic criterion; it is just an epidemiological data. However, during anamnesis, the patient with hypnic headache should be asked about this characteristic of pain, as several authors describe the headache as dull or pressure quality [8, 9, 23].

In the review of 345 patients with hypnic headache, in 74.4% of the cases, the pain had a dull or pressure quality; throbbing or pulsatile, in 18.3%; and stabbing or burning, in 7.3%. In some cases, patients described pain as non-pulsatile, but in practice it was considered dull or pressure [2–4].

Pain Intensity

Although pain intensity is not a diagnostic criterion for hypnic headache, ICHD-3 adds in its final comments that pain is generally mild to moderate in intensity; however, severe pain is reported by 20% of patients [1].

The quantification of the painful experience is done through verbal descriptors that represent different subjective intensities of pain, such as mild, moderate, intense, or very intense. Usually, the visual analogue scale (VAS) is used to assist the patient. This scale consists of numbering from zero (no pain) to ten (maximum pain). According to VAS, we will have the following verbal descriptors: mild (VAS 1–4), moderate (VAS 5–7), severe (VAS 8–9), and very severe (VAS 10). There will be no pain when VAS equals zero.

In the review of 345 patients with hypnic headache, in 61.5% of them, the pain intensity was moderate; in 32.5%, it was severe; and in 0.8%, very severe. Pain was mild in only 5.5% and, in this case, the patient was able to fall asleep again, regardless of the duration of the pain [2–4].

Pain Location

Pain location in hypnic headache patients is discussed since the initial proposal of their diagnostic criteria. Initially, it was not known whether the pain was unilateral or bilateral. However, the cases published in the last 34 years have shown that it is mainly bilateral. Pain location is not a diagnostic criterion, but, in the final comments of ICHD-3, it is added that pain is bilateral in about two-thirds of cases [1].

In the review of 345 patients with hypnic headache, in 55.5% of them, the pain was bilateral; in 30.3%, it was unilateral; and in 14.2%, it was holocranial (diffuse). In cases where the pain was unilateral, there was a predominance of the left side (57.8%), typically frontotemporal [2–4].

Associated Symptoms

As soon as the first suggestions for diagnostic criteria for hypnic headache appeared, it was believed that the patient could not have manifestations associated with headache, such as nausea, photophobia, and phonophobia [24]. After inclusion of hypnic headache in ICHD-2, it was determined that there could be no more than one of the following symptoms: nausea, photophobia, or phonophobia [25].

In the review of 345 patients with hypnic headache, most patients (62.6%) did not have any manifestations associated with headache. Nausea and / or vomiting were present in 21.9% of patients; photophobia or phonophobia, in 11.9%; and photophobia and phonophobia, in 3.6%. Nausea alone was the main manifestation associated with headache attacks, occurring in 21% of cases. No patient with hypnic headache had any kind of aura preceding or accompanying the headache attacks [2–4].

Although the characteristics of hypnic headache are generally similar to tension-type headache, recent studies have shown that many patients could experience nausea during attacks, similar to migraine [1].

Autonomic Manifestations

In the first hypnic headache patients described by Raskin in 1988, none of them had any autonomic manifestations associated with headache [18]. From the first diagnostic criteria, it was quite clear that pain is not associated with autonomic signs and/or symptoms. [23, 24] According to ICHD-3, for the diagnosis of hypnic headache, the absence of cranial autonomic symptoms or restlessness is necessary [1].

However, from the publications of case reports on hypnic headache, it was found that some patients had autonomic symptoms that met diagnostic criteria for cluster headache or chronic paroxysmal hemicrania, although none of these patients met the complete criteria for trigeminal autonomic cephalalgias [6].

In the review of 345 patients with hypnic headache, autonomic manifestations were present in 7.6% of patients with hypnic headache, with a predominance of tearing (61.1%) and rhinorrhea (16.7%) [2–4]. Usually, when autonomic manifestations were present, they were mild and bilaterally located [21, 24].

Triggering Factors

In most primary headaches, there is a trigger for the onset of headache attacks. In the case of hypnic headache, sleep is recognized as the main trigger because headache attacks occur exclusively during sleep. However, the most studied trigger for hypnic headache is drinking alcohol.

In the first cases described, alcohol ingestion had no influence on headache attacks [18], but it is already known that patients with hypnic headache may have headache attacks triggered by drinking alcohol the night before [7, 28].

References

1. Headache Classification Subcommittee of the International Headache Society. The International Classification of Headache Disorders, 3rd edition. Cephalalgia. 2018;38(1):1–211.
2. Silva-Néto RP, Sousa-Santos PEM, Peres MFP. Hypnic headache: a review of 348 cases published from 1988 to 2018. J Neurol Sci. 2019;401:103–9.
3. Zhang Y, Wang C, Chen Y, Wang R, Lian Y. Hypnic headache with dopaminergic neuron dysfunction: new insight from a rare case. Pain Med. 2019;20(8):1639–42.
4. Kesserwani H. Hypnic headache responds to topiramate: a case report and a review of mechanisms of action of therapeutic agents. Cureus. 2021;13(3):e13790.
5. Silva-Néto RP, Almeida KJ. Hypnic headache: a descriptive study of 25 new cases in Brazil. J Neurol Sci. 2014;338(1–2):166–8.
6. Evers S, Goadsby PJ. Hypnic headache. Pract Neurol. 2005;5(3):144–9.
7. Pinto CAR, Fragoso YD, Souza Carvalho D, Gabbai AA. Síndrome da cefaleia hípnica: aspectos clínicos de 16 pacientes. Rev Neurociênc. 2003;11(1):46–51.
8. Dodick DW, Mosek AC, Campbell JK. The hypnic ('alarm clock') headache syndrome. Cephalalgia. 1998;18(3):152–6.

9. Klimek A, Sklodowski P, Night headache. Report of 2 cases. Neurol Neurochir Pol. 1999;33(5):49–54.
10. Casucci G. Chronic short-lasting headaches: clinical features and differential diagnosis. Neurol Sci. 2003;24(2):101–7.
11. Escudero Martínez I, González-Oria C, Bernal Sánchez-Arjona M, Jiménez Hernández MD. Description of series of 10 patients with hypnic headache: discussion of the diagnostic criteria. Neurologia. 2015;30(4):195–200.
12. Liang JF, Fuh JL, Yu HY, Hsu CY, Wang SJ. Clinical features, polysomnography and outcome in patients with hypnic headache. Cephalalgia. 2008;28(3):209–15.
13. Prakash S, Dahbi AS. Relapsing remitting hypnic headache responsive to indomethacin in an adolescent: a case report. J Headache Pain. 2008;9(6):393–5.
14. Dolso P, Merlino G, Fratticci L, Canesin R, Valiante G, Coccolo D, et al. Non-REM hypnic headache: a circadian disorder? A clinical and polysomnography. Cephalalgia. 2006;27(1):83–6.
15. Pinessi L, Rainero I, Cicolin A, Zibetti M, Gentile S, Mutani R. Hypnic headache syndrome: association of the attacks with REM sleep. Cephalalgia. 2003;23(2):150–4.
16. Ghiotto N, Sances G, Di Lorenzo G, Trucco M, Loi M, Sandrini G, et al. Report of eight new cases of hypnic headache and mini-review of the literature. Funct Neurol. 2002;17(4):211–9.
17. Pinto CAR, Fragoso YD, Souza Carvalho D, Gabbai AA. Hypnic headache syndrome: clinical aspects of eight patients in Brazil. Cephalalgia. 2002;22(10):824–7.
18. Raskin NH. The hypnic headache syndrome. Headache. 1988;28(8):534–6.
19. Relja G, Zorzon M, Locatelli L, Carraro N, Antonello RM, Cazzato G. Hypnic headache: rapid and long-lasting response to prednisone in two new cases. Cephalalgia. 2002;22(2):157–9.
20. Queiroz LP, Coral LC. The hypnic headache syndrome – a case report (Abstract). Proceedings of 8th Congress of the International Headache Society, 1997 Jun 10–14; Amsterdam, Germany. Cephalalgia. 1997;17(3):303.
21. Lisoto C, Mainardi F, Maggioni F, Zanchin G. Episodic hypnic headache? Cephalalgia. 2004;24(8):681–5.
22. Evers S, Rahmann A, Schwaag S, Lüdermann P, Husstedt IW. Hypnic headache – the first German cases including polysomnography. Cephalalgia. 2003;23(1):20–3.
23. Goadsby PJ, Lipton RB. A review of paroxysmal hemicranias, SUNCT syndrome and other short-lasting headaches with autonomic feature, including new cases. Brain. 1997;120(1):193–209.
24. Evers S, Goadsby PJ. Hypnic headache: clinical features, pathophysiology, and treatment. Neurology. 2003;60(6):905–9.
25. Headache Classification Subcommittee of the International Headache Society. The international classification of headache disorders, 2nd edition. Cephalalgia. 2004;24(1):8–160.
26. Gil-Gouveia R, Goadsby PJ. Secondary hypnic headache. J Neurol. 2007;254(5):646–54.
27. Sandrini G, Tassorelli C, Ghiotto N, Nappi G. Uncommon primary headaches. Curr Opin Neurol. 2006;19(3):299–304.
28. Dodick DW, Jones JM, Capobianco DJ. Hypnic headache: another indomethacin-responsive headache syndrome? Headache. 2000;40(10):830–5.

Chapter 6
Clinical Characteristics in Children

Nothing makes us as big as great pain

Alfred Musset (1810–1857)

Introduction

Headache is a common complaint in pediatric age. At this age, the diagnosis of migraine and/or tension-type headache is very common. Other primary headaches appear to be extremely rare and often unidentified or underdiagnosed by the pediatrician.

Hypnic headache is one of the rare headaches. According to five studies conducted at tertiary headache centers in different countries, its prevalence was estimated at 0.07–0.35% of all headache patients [1–5]. In children, it is much more rare. In June 2019, the most recent literature review on hypnic headache was published, in which 343 adult patients and only five children with this headache were described [6].

This headache has been widely studied and well defined in the adult population. This is due to the almost exclusive predominance in adults and the onset of pain after 50 years of age. A recent review on hypnic headache in adults showed that the mean age of headache onset was 58 years, ranging from 15 to 85 years [6].

The first description of this headache was made in adults aged ≥65 years [7]. From there, with the description of new cases, diagnostic criteria were elaborated, resulting in their inclusion in ICHD-2. However, in this classification, a diagnostic criterion establishes that headache must occur for the first time after 50 years of age (See Table 2.5 in Chap. 2) [8].

R. Silva-Néto, D. Holle-Lee, *Hypnic Headache*,
https://doi.org/10.1007/978-3-031-32263-1_6

Diagnostic Criteria

After the publication of ICHD-2, there were reports of cases of hypnic headache in childhood [9–11], contradicting one of its characteristics, which would be the occurrence, for the first time, after 50 years of age [8].

In the diagnostic criteria of ICHD-3, hypnic headache is not exclusive to any age group. It is characterized by the presence of recurrent headache episodes that, in addition to appearing only during sleep and causing the patient to awaken, occur for 10 or more days per month, for more than 3 months, lasting more than 15 mins, for up to 4 h after awakening and without autonomic symptoms or restlessness (Table 6.1) [12].

Currently, the few cases reported in childhood [9–11] indicate that one should look carefully for the neglected diagnosis of hypnic headache and reconsider its authenticity and mechanism in childhood.

Table 6.1 Diagnostic criteria for ICHD-3 for hypnic headache (2018)

A. Recurrent headache attacks fulfilling criteria B–E
B. Developing only during sleep, and causing wakening
C. Occurring on ≥10 days/month for >3 months
D. Lasting from 15 mins up to 4 h after waking
E. No cranial autonomic symptoms or restlessness.
F. Not better accounted for by another ICHD-3 diagnosis

Epidemiological Data

From 1988 to 2022, only five children (three girls and two boys) were diagnosed with hypnic headache [9–11]. Clinical and demographic characteristics of these children, which are summarized in Table 6.2, were based on a recently published review article on hypnic headache in childhood [13].

Table 6.2 Demographic and clinical characteristics of five children with hypnic headache

	Cases reported				
Characteristics	Grosberg et al.(2004)	Scagni et al. (2008)	Cerminara et al. (2011)		
Sex	F	F	M	M	F
Age (years)	9	8	7	11	10
Pre-diagnostic disease duration (months)	2	60	6	1	10
Time of occurrence	1–2 a.m. (5–6 h after falling asleep)	2–4 a.m.	1–3 h after falling asleep	1–2 a.m. and 4–5 a.m.	1–2 h after falling asleep
Duration of attacks (min)	30	30–60	20–30	10–20	10–30
Able to return to sleep after relief of pain	Yes	Yes	Yes	Yes	Yes
Wake painless in the morning	Yes	Yes	NI	NI	NI
Number of attacks per night	1	1	NI	2–3	2–3
Frequency (days/month)	8–12	1	2	20–25	10–15
Intensity of pain	Moderate to severe	Severe	Moderate	Moderate to severe	Moderate to severe
Character of pain	Throbbing	Pulsating	NI	Dull	Pulsating
Concomitant symptoms (nausea, photophobia, or phonophobia	Absent	Absent	Absent	Occasionally nausea	Occasionally nausea
Autonomic symptoms	Absent	Absent	Absent	Absent	Absent
Side of pain	Unilateral	Bilateral	Bilateral	Bilateral	Bilateral
Localization	Right frontal and temporal	Frontal	Frontal-temporal	Frontal-temporal	Frontal or frontal-temporal
General/neurologic exam	Normal	Normal	Normal	Normal	Normal

(continued)

Table 6.2 (continued)

Characteristics	Cases reported				
	Grosberg et al.(2004)	Scagni et al. (2008)	Cerminara et al. (2011)		
Routine blood tests (biochemical and hematological)	Normal	Normal	Normal	Blood iron 144 mg/dL (35–140) and ferritin 1928 ng/mL (13–150)	Normal
Brain MRI and EEG	Normal	Normal	Normal	Normal	Normal
Comorbidities	Absent	Absent	Absent	Thalassemia major	Absent
Family history of headache	NI	Positive	Positive (mother has migraine without aura)	Negative	Negative
Abortive medication	No	Acetaminophen	No	No	No
Preventive medication	No	No	No	Melatonin	Melatonin
Total follow time (months)	2	12	12	6	3

F: female; M: male; NI: No Information.
Source: Silva-Néto RP, Almeida KJ. Hypnic headache in childhood: A literature review. J Neurol Sci 2015;356 (1, 2):45–8

The mean age of the patients was 9.0 ± 1.6 years (95%CI 7.6–10.4), ranging from 7 to 11 years. In no case was there a family history of hypnic headache, but a positive history for other primary headaches in two patients [9–10]. Mother of one of them had migraine without aura [9].

Disease Duration until Diagnosis

The diagnosis was made, on average, 15.8 months (ranging from 1 to 60 months) after the onset of headache, showing that this condition is still little recognized and, therefore, underdiagnosed [13].

Time of Onset of Pain

Hypnic headache, by definition, appears only during sleep and causes the patient to awaken [12]. All children who had this diagnosis were awakened by pain during nighttime sleep but were able to go back to sleep after pain relief. They woke up without pain the next morning [9–11, 13].

Most patients were awakened by pain a few hours after falling asleep and the time of onset of pain was between one and three in the morning [13].

Duration of Headache Attacks

No patient had a headache lasting more than an hour. In four of them (80%), the duration of the headache was approximately 10–30 mins; and in just one, the pain lasted up to 60 mins [13]. According to the current diagnostic criteria for hypnic headache, the duration of pain, after awakening, is ≥15 mins and disappears within 4 h [12].

Frequency of Headache Attacks

Frequency of headache attacks varied from one to three episodes per night, but less than 15 days of headache occurred in each month in 80% of patients. Among the characteristics of hypnic headache, the frequency of pain is 10 or more days per month, for more than 3 months [12]. However, several authors, when studying adult patients, reported a high frequency of attacks on more than 15 days per month [14–16] and, in some cases, up to three times a night [16–17].

Quality of Pain

In adults with hypnic headache, many authors have described the quality or character of pain as dull or pressure [5, 16, 18], but a review of 94 patients showed 57% of them having a dull character and in 39% the pain was throbbing [16].

During the review of pediatric cases, it was found that pain was described as pulsating or throbbing, in 60% of cases [13]. However, it is good to remember that in none of the classifications, the quality of pain was or is a diagnostic criterion for hypnic headache [8, 12].

Pain Intensity

All children were able to report the intensity of the pain and described it as being moderate to severe. Exclusively in those who received prophylactic treatment, there was a decrease in intensity and the pain that was severe decreased to moderate [13].

It seems that the pain is more severe in children, as reviews of hypnic headache in adults have shown that the intensity of the pain, for the most part, is mild to moderate [5, 6, 16].

Pain Location

Of the five children with hypnic headache, four reported pain in the frontal and/or temporal region, in which the main location was bilateral. In only one child, the pain was unilateral on the right [13]. The involvement of the frontotemporal region is also typical in adults, including the periorbital region [16].

Since the initial proposal for the diagnostic criteria for hypnic headache, the topographic location of pain is discussed [19]. Subsequent publications showed that the location of pain is predominantly bilateral [5, 6, 16, 20].

Concomitant Symptoms

In some primary headaches, there is an association with other signs and/or symptoms. In migraine, for example, the presence of nausea, vomiting, photophobia, and phonophobia are diagnostic criteria; and in trigeminal autonomic cephalalgias, the following parasympathetic autonomic manifestations are observed ipsilateral to the headache: conjunctival hyperemia, tearing, nasal congestion, rhinorrhea, frontal and facial sweating, myosis and ptosis, and edema of the eyelid [12].

In order to avoid diagnostic confusion, as soon as the first cases of hypnic headache were described, even before their inclusion in the classification of headache, the differential diagnosis was immediately made with migraine and trigeminal autonomic cephalalgias. Thus, the patient could not have any of the associated manifestations that were mentioned above, even if there was an aggravation of the headache with routine physical activities [19].

When the hypnic headache was included in ICHD-2, criterion D stated that there should be "absence of autonomic signs and presence of no more than one of the following symptoms: nausea, photophobia or phonophobia." [8] In ICHD-3, it is only necessary that there are no cranial autonomic symptoms or restlessness [12].

In the children described with hypnic headache, none reported vomiting, photophobia, phonophobia, or any autonomic symptoms associated with headache attacks, but two of them occasionally had nausea [1, 9].

The classic symptoms associated with migraine headache have been described in a few adult patients with hypnic headache [5, 6, 17, 21]. In a review of 94 cases of hypnic headache, nausea was a complaint in 22% of patients; and vomiting, in none. Photophobia or phonophobia, both of mild intensity were cited by 5% of patients [16].

Complementary Exams

Hypnic headache is a primary disorder of the central nervous system. Therefore, it is not attributed to another disease and is not better explained by another diagnosis of the current classification of headache [12]. Neuroimaging tests are only used to exclude secondary headaches and not to confirm hypnic headache.

In all children with this headache, the neurological examination was normal. Complementary exams performed were brain MRI and sleep-deprived EEG, which were also normal [13]. Laboratory investigation (biochemistry and blood count) was changed only in one patient who had thalassemia major [9].

Comorbidities

No child reported a previous history of headache. All children were healthy, except for one who had thalassemia major and had undergone a bone marrow transplant 6 months before the onset of pain. In this child, his drug treatment included cyclosporine, methylprednisolone, amoxicillin, fluconazole, and acyclovir [9].

Treatment and Follow-Up

Acute and prophylactic treatments of hypnic headache in childhood are made according to the reports or case series of adult patients. However, none of these studies have been controlled. Thus, treatment recommendations are based on observational studies and need validation.

The five pediatric cases, treated or untreated, were followed, after diagnosis, for a period of 7.0 ± 4.8 months (95% CI 2.8–11.2), ranging from 2 to 12 months [9–11, 13].

Acute Treatment

According to ICHD-3, recurrent episodes of hypnic headache last up to 4 h and often do not require treatment [12]. In the published pediatric cases, the majority of patients (80%) did not take any medication because each headache attack was completely relieved in about 30 mins. Only one patient used symptomatic medication (paracetamol) which provided relief in approximately 30–60 mins [10].

Prophylactic Treatment

Of the five children with hypnic headache, one had spontaneous remission 2 months after diagnosis [11], and in two, the headache attacks persisted for more than a year, with no change in frequency or intensity. They did not undergo any prophylactic treatment, due to the low frequency of headache attacks [9, 10]. Only two children were treated prophylactically and used melatonin [9].

In the first one that used melatonin, the initial dose was 2 mg/day, at bedtime. There was a reduction in the intensity (severe pain reduced to moderate pain) and frequency (25–30 attacks per month reduced to 10–15 attacks per month) of headache attacks. The dose was increased to 4 mg / day and this child became asymptomatic for a period of 6 months [9].

In the second child, the initial dose of melatonin was 3 mg/day, at bedtime. There was a reduction in the intensity (severe pain reduced to moderate pain) and frequency (12–15 attacks per month reduced to 1–2 attacks per month) of headache attacks. In the following 2 months, this child remained asymptomatic [9].

Conclusions

Hypnic headache is a rare disorder that usually occurs, for the first time, in the elderly, but it can start in childhood with the same characteristics as adults.

References

1. Silva-Néto RP, Almeida KJ. Hypnic headache: a descriptive study of 25 new cases in Brazil. J Neurol Sci. 2014;338(1–2):166–8.
2. Donnet A, Lantéri-Minet M. A consecutive series of 22 cases of hypnic headache in France. Cephalalgia. 2009;29(9):928–34.
3. Liang JF, Fuh JL, Yu HY, Hsu CY, Wang SJ. Clinical features, polysomnography and outcome in patients with hypnic headache. Cephalalgia. 2008;28(3):209–15.
4. Lisoto C, Mainardi F, Maggioni F, Zanchin G. Episodic hypnic headache? Cephalalgia. 2004;24(8):681–5.
5. Dodick DW, Mosek AC, Campbell JK. The hypnic ('alarm clock') headache syndrome. Cephalalgia. 1998;18(3):152–6.
6. Silva-Néto RP, Sousa-Santos PEM, Peres MFP. Hypnic headache: a review of 348 cases published from 1988 to 2018. J Neurol Sci. 2019;401:103–9.
7. Raskin NH. The hypnic headache syndrome. Headache. 1988;28(8):534–6.
8. Headache Classification Subcommittee of the International Headache Society. The international classification of headache disorders, 2nd edition. Cephalalgia. 2004;24(1):8–160.
9. Cerminara C, Compagnone E, Coniglio A, Margiotta M, Curatolo P, Villa MP, et al. Hypnic headache in children. Cephalalgia. 2011;31(16):1673–6.
10. Scagni P, Pagliero R. Hypnic in childhood: a new report. J Paediatr Child Health. 2008;44(1–2):83–4.

11. Grosberg BM, Lipton RB, Solomon S, Ballaban-Gil K. Hypnic headache in childhood? A case report. Cephalalgia. 2004;25(1):68–70.
12. Headache Classification Subcommittee of the International Headache Society. The international classification of headache disorders, 3rd edition. Cephalalgia. 2018;38(1):1–211.
13. Silva-Néto RP, Almeida KJ. Hypnic headache in childhood: a literature review. J Neurol Sci. 2015;356(1–2):45–8.
14. Gil-Gouveia R, Goadsby PJ. Secondary hypnic headache. J Neurol. 2007;254(5):646–54.
15. Sandrini G, Tassorelli C, Ghiotto N, Nappi G. Uncommon primary headaches. Curr Opin Neurol. 2006;19(3):299–304.
16. Evers S, Goadsby PJ. Hypnic headache. Pract Neurol. 2005;5(3):144–9.
17. Casucci G. Chronic short-lasting headaches: clinical features and differential diagnosis. Neurol Sci. 2003;24(2):101–7.
18. Klimek A, Sklodowski P, Night headache. Report of 2 cases. Neurol Neurochir Pol. 1999;33(5):49–54.
19. Goadsby PJ, Lipton RB. A review of paroxysmal hemicranias, SUNCT syndrome and other short-lasting headaches with autonomic feature, including new cases. Brain. 1997;120(1):193–209.
20. Pinto CAR, Fragoso YD, Souza Carvalho D, Gabbai AA. Síndrome da cefaleia hípnica: aspectos clínicos de 16 pacientes. Rev Neurociênc. 2003;11(1):46–51.
21. Newman LC, Lipton RB, Solomon S. The hypnic headache syndrome: a benign headache disorder of the elderly. Neurology. 1990;40(12):1904–5.

Chapter 7
Pathophysiology

The art of medicine is to distract the patient while Nature takes care of the disease

Voltaire (1694–1778)

Introduction

Pathophysiology of hypnic headache is unknown to many researchers [1–3]. Its exact pathophysiological mechanism has not been elucidated yet [4]. There are only speculations, considering that the studies are not experimental [5, 6].

Some hypotheses suggest that hypnic headache results from disturbed REM (rapid eye movement) sleep, chronobiological disorder, or deregulation of serotonin and melatonin [6–14]. An important pathophysiological mechanism is the association with hypothalamic dysfunction [15].

Headache and Sleep

Headaches and sleep disorders are common complaints in neurological practice. If the two complaints are associated, they will be responsible for numerous social and family problems, leading to a major socio-economic impact.

For over a century, researchers have known the relationship between headache and sleep [16]. Headache can occur during sleep, in any of its phases. It can also be triggered by deprivation or excessive sleep [13]. It was observed that in the REM stage of sleep, pain of greater intensity and duration is required to wake the individual from ongoing sleep inhibitory mechanisms [17].

Headache attacks during sleep occur in hypnic headache, in other primary headaches (migraine and trigeminal-autonomic cephalalgia) and in several headaches

R. Silva-Néto, D. Holle-Lee, *Hypnic Headache*,
https://doi.org/10.1007/978-3-031-32263-1_7

secondary, such as sleep apnea, giant cell arteritis, intracranial hypertension due to hydrocephalus and intracranial neoplasia [13, 18, 19].

It is questioned whether hypnic headache is a subtype of cluster headache. However, the only feature that supports this hypothesis is the occurrence of pain during sleep. In hypnic headache, pain is not strictly unilateral, nor is parasympathetic activation required, as is generally observed in trigeminal-autonomic cephalalgias. It is worth mentioning that some cases of cluster headache would fulfill diagnostic criteria for hypnic headache, if the presence of autonomic symptoms was omitted from these criteria [5, 6].

Some researchers argue that hypnic headache is a sleep disorder, much more than a primary headache. Interestingly, a patient with hypnic headache had remission of the headache attacks for 3 months after traveling in all time zones [20].

Hypnic Headache and REM Sleep

The occurrence of sleep-related headache attacks is a characteristic of hypnic headache. Since its initial description, it has been tried to relate it to a sleep disorder. In that description, it was observed that some patients woke up with headache during dreams [21]. For this reason, it was concluded that REM sleep was an important factor in the generation of hypnic headache and that it would be the paradigm of a headache that appears during dreams [13].

As soon as the first cases of hypnic headache were described, it was suggested, and even demonstrated by polysomnographic studies, that this headache would be a REM sleep disorder, as headache attacks occurred in this phase of sleep [6–9, 11, 22, 23].

It was believed that the functions of the raphe nuclei, the locus cœruleus and the periaqueductal gray substance, which are essential parts of the anti-nociceptive system, were impaired during REM sleep [12, 24, 25].

Some authors stated that the hypnic headache could be due to arterial hypertension and low oxygenation that occur during REM sleep. This condition has been called nocturnal headache syndrome and hypertension and could be successfully treated with antihypertensive medication [12, 26].

Despite the strong relationship between headache and REM sleep, this assumption has been questioned in recent publications. There is evidence that most attacks of hypnic headache arise in non-REM sleep, especially in stages 2 and 3 [27, 28]. However, a more detailed analysis did not reveal a subtype of hypnic headache in REM or non-REM sleep, since the headache can be detected in both phases of sleep, in the same patient and on the same night [29].

It appears that the association between REM sleep and hypnic headache may not be specific, as there is a frequent onset of headache attacks during REM sleep in patients with migraine and episodic cluster headache [5, 6]. Perhaps the pathophysiological correlate of hypnic headache is in microstructural changes in sleep [30].

Polysomnography

In hypnic headache, headache attacks occur during sleep and awaken the patient. They can last up to 4 hours after awakening [31]. Morning or nocturnal headache is one of the clinical manifestations of different types of sleep apnea, therefore, patients with hypnic headache need to undergo polysomnographic studies [32, 33]. Furthermore, there is some evidence that hypnic headache is related to REM sleep [6].

Patients with hypnic headache underwent polysomnography in a study. None of them had obstructive sleep apnea syndrome or another type of nocturnal deoxygenation [32]. In another study, three patients had evidence of hypnic headache attacks always occurring during the REM sleep stage. They underwent overnight polysomnography. In all three patients, the headache attacks occurred during the first REM stage. In a single patient, the headache attack was recorded during a time of oxygen desaturation. This patient improved after oxygen supplementation with continuous positive airway pressure (CPAP) [12].

A 79-year-old woman diagnosed with hypnic headache underwent a polysomnographic study, which showed awakening at stage 3 slow wave sleep because of a nocturnal headache attack. Although this finding could be nonspecific, it suggests a possible relationship between stage 3 slow wave sleep and hypnic headache [28].

A polysomnographic study was performed on three patients with hypnic headache. Headache attacks occurred in only two of them, always during the first stage of REM sleep, with a decrease in the mean nocturnal oxygen saturation, but without apnea. No patient improved with nocturnal oxygen inhalation. In one of the patients, the headache attack was associated with periodic movements of the legs throughout the night without awakening [10].

Since the first cases of hypnic headache described by Raskin, it has been known that headache attacks can occur during dreams [21]. Polysomnographic studies may show headache attacks during dreams, both in nightmares and in vivid dreams [6]. Despite the relationship between headache and dreaming, no formal evaluation of dreams with nocturnal polysomnography has been reported for this syndrome. Of the 345 adult patients with hypnic headache that have been described, in two of them the headache attacks came on during a nightmare [34, 35]; and 10 patients, during vivid dreams [3, 10, 11, 34, 36–38].

In the literature review, it was found that 23 polysomnography were performed in 101 patients diagnosed with hypnic headache. In most patients, there was a decrease in sleep quality. In one patient, there was severe obstructive sleep apnea; in 14, onset of headache during sleep (in 10 of them during REM sleep, and in four, during stages 2 or 3 of non-REM sleep); and in 4, it was totally normal [1, 6, 9, 12, 22, 28, 39]. Patients who did not undergo polysomnography reported that their headache attacks started during dreams or nightmares [5].

A polysomnographic study was carried out in nine hypnic headache patients, without using specific medication for a period of 7 days preceding the examination.

The following parameters were analyzed during sleep: sleep stage and efficiency, apneas and hypopneas, arousals and micro-arousals, cardiac events, oxyhemoglobin saturation, and limb movements [40].

In this study, polysomnography revealed poor sleep efficiency in seven patients; increase in the number of micro-awakenings, in seven; decreased REM sleep, in six; absence of REM sleep, in one; mild obstructive apneas, in six; and snoring, in three [40]. Possibly, these findings justify the frequent complaint of non-restorative sleep in hypnic headache patients.

Unfortunately, polysomnographic studies are not routinely performed in patients diagnosed with hypnic headache. According to the authors, a thorough sleep assessment should be performed in all patients with hypnic headache. This conduct would have pathophysiological and therapeutic implications for this disease.

Chronobiological Disorder and Dysregulation of Serotonin and Melatonin

Hypnic headache is believed to be a chronobiological disorder because many patients experience headache attacks always at the same time during the night, hence the name "alarm clock headache." [3]

In the pathophysiology of hypnic headache, there seems to be a pacemaker or biological clock mechanism [13]. By the way, the brain structure recognized as this pacemaker is the suprachiasmatic nucleus (SCN), one of the most important biological clocks that control circadian rhythm (from Latin circa, around; and *diem*, day) and the cycle daily endogenous.

This nucleus consists of two small cell groups located in the anterior part of the hypothalamus and above the optical chiasm. It has afferent and efferent projections to the periaqueductal gray and aminergic nuclei, which are the most important structures of the brain stem for pain modulation [6, 13, 23, 41, 42].

Neurodegenerative pathogenicity of hypnic headache is suspected, due to its predominance in the sixth and seventh decades of life. There is cell loss with aging; consequently, there is a decrease in the activity of the hypothalamic–pineal axis, particularly the SCN. This nucleus maintains a close relationship of neighborhood and function with the pineal gland, with that, there will be a decrease or absence of melatonin secretion [6, 13, 23, 41–43]

Melatonin is a neurohormone synthesized and secreted by the pineal gland mainly during the night. Melatonin secretion is regulated by the hypothalamus, notably by the SCN. A lack of melatonin and cortisol rhythmicity was also seen in patients with cluster headache but there is still no data for hypnic headache [44]. The exact pathophysiological mechanism of melatonin is still unknown. Analgesic effects have been suggested, including potentiation of GABAergic inhibition, as well as modulation of cellular calcium influx and modulation of 5HT2 receptors

[43]. It is believed that the aging of the suprachiasmatic nucleus explains why many patients respond to melatonin [45].

Melatonin would have several physiological functions, such as, for example, modulation of the gabaergic system in nociceptive circuits, control of cerebral vascular tone, facilitation of neurotransmission mediated by 5-HT_2 receptors and production of mediators involved in inflammation, such as prostaglandin E_2. This could explain how the decrease in melatonin secretion would cause the development of hypnic headache [3, 13] and its exogenous administration would cause an improvement [12].

Hypothalamus has a great influence on hypnic headache. It is considered an important center of integration and regulation of the nervous and endocrine systems. An example of this is the timing of hypnic headache attacks and the concomitant diabetes insipidus with a feeling of intense thirst, favoring the involvement of hypothalamic structures [46]. Hypothalamus acts on pain control and sleep regulation. This mechanism is consequent to its strong connections with the periaqueductal gray matter, locus coeruleus, and raphe nuclei [47]. In addition, hypothalamus maintains connections with the caudal trigeminal nucleus through the trigeminal-hypothalamic tract [48].

In mammals, the biological clock is modulated by serotonin. This would explain how lithium, which increases serotonergic neurotransmission in the hypothalamus, would be useful in the treatment of hypnic headache and also other chronobiological disorders, such as cluster headache, nocturnal migraine, and affective disorders [13].

This serotonergic neurotransmission in the hypothalamus occurs due to lithium's ability to affect serotonin metabolism by increasing its release and deregulation of its receptors [49]. In addition, lithium indirectly increases the level of melatonin [50–52] and therefore interferes with the pathophysiology of hypnic headache.

In addition to the mechanisms already discussed above, the possibility that the pathophysiology is heterogeneous is also questioned, due to the differences in polysomnographic studies and the variety of drugs reported as effective in the treatment of hypnic headache. Further investigations using functional neuroimaging studies are necessary to better understand its pathophysiology [4].

A few years ago, it was claimed that structural injuries or metabolic dysfunction that occurred in hypnic headache could not yet be detected. Therefore, this headache was not classified as symptomatic; and yes, idiopathic, even though there is no evidence of a genetic predisposition, probably due to the small number of published cases. On the other hand, the exclusion of symptomatic headache depends on systematic studies on metabolic changes or other underlying sleep disorders [5, 6].

There is an investigation by neuroimaging that used voxel-based morphometry (a neologism that mixes the words "volume" and "pixel") to analyze structural changes, comparing patients with hypnic headache to healthy controls. A significant reduction in the gray matter in the posterior hypothalamus of hypnic headache patients has been shown [29]. It is in this region of the brain where the human biological clock is located. This observation was the first pathophysiological correlation of hypothalamic dysfunction in hypnic headache [27]. Although hypothalamic changes are not specific for hypnic headache, these findings may lead to future research.

Hypnic Headache and Caffeine

The role of caffeine as an adjunct in pain treatment is controversial. Potential mechanism of caffeine as an analgesic are uncertain. More large-scale high-quality studies are needed to demonstrate its effectiveness. Different mechanisms of caffeine in pain regulation are studied [53].

First, by blocking the action of adenosine, it becomes a potent cerebral vasoconstrictor [54] and, due to its effectiveness in hypnic headache, it is suggested the involvement of the vascular system and/or alteration of the level of excitability in its pathophysiology [29].

Another mechanism demonstrated in studies is the anti-nociceptive effect of caffeine, which seems to result from its interaction with adenosine receptors. These receptors are divided into four subtypes in the human body: A_1, A_{2A}, A_{2B}, and A_3, expressed in different areas of the central and peripheral nervous system [53, 54]. In neuropathic pain, nociceptive, and inflammatory models, activation of A_1 and A_{2A} receptors results in antinociception [55, 56]. It is possible that hypnic headache patients have a different adenosine receptor profiles [46].

There is also a potential effect of caffeine on sleep. It influences sleep induction through A_{2a} brain adenosine receptors [57]. Caffeine-induced wakefulness is mainly based on the antagonism of this receptor. The structure of caffeine is similar to that of adenosine; hence it competes with it for A_{2A} receptors, leading them to be inhibited [58]. However, hypnic headache patients, for unknown reasons, do not report difficulties in inducing sleep after drinking coffee before bed or during headache attacks [46].

Possibly, the good therapeutic response to caffeine provides information about the pathophysiology of hypnic headache. Many patients report a good therapeutic effect of caffeine associated with painkillers; but not, of painkillers alone. It is recommended to drink a cup of coffee both during headache attacks and in their prevention [27, 46, 59]. However, a randomized clinical trial is still required to verify its effectiveness.

Hypnic Headache and Indomethacin

Indomethacin, a non-steroidal anti-inflammatory (NSAID), has potent inhibitory effects on the synthesis of prostaglandins. At a dose between 25 and 150 mg/day, it showed a good therapeutic response in the prophylactic treatment of hypnic headache [59].

This anti-inflammatory has some distinct properties that differentiate it from other NSAIDs, which may explain why there are headaches responsive to indomethacin [59], such as, for example, paroxysmal hemicrania, continuous hemicrania, primary headache, primary cough headache, and primary stress headache [60].

Indomethacin crosses the blood–brain barrier better than naproxen and ibuprofen [60], suggesting a central action in the treatment of headache [61]. Experimental studies have shown that indomethacin inhibits nitric oxide-induced dural vasodilation, whose role in the pathophysiology of headache is crucial. On the other hand, naproxen and ibuprofen did not reduce this vasodilation [61].

It is believed that there are direct and indirect mechanisms, among them, the second messenger, involved in the effects of nitric oxide in headache and specific subtypes of these mechanisms that can differentiate several primary headaches sensitive to indomethacin, such as hypnic headache [46, 62].

References

1. Gil-Gouveia R, Goadsby PJ. Secondary hypnic headache. J Neurol. 2007;254(5):646–54.
2. Klimek A, Sklodowski P, Night headache. Report of 2 cases. Neurol Neurochir Pol. 1999;33(5):49–54.
3. Dodick DW, Mosek AC, Campbell JK. The hypnic ('alarm clock') headache syndrome. Cephalalgia. 1998;18(3):152–6.
4. Lisotto C, Rossi P, Tassorelli C, Ferrante E, Nappi G. Focus on therapy of hypnic headache. J Headache Pain. 2010;11(4):349–54.
5. Evers S, Goadsby PJ. Hypnic headache. Pract Neurol. 2005;5(3):144–9.
6. Evers S, Goadsby PJ. Hypnic headache: clinical features, pathophysiology, and treatment. Neurology. 2003;60(6):905–9.
7. Seidel S, Zeitlhofer J, Wöber C. First Austrian case of hypnic headache: serial polysomnography and blood pressure monitoring in treatment with indomethacin. Cephalalgia. 2008;28(10):1086–90.
8. Peters N, Lorenzl S, Fischereder J, Bötzel K, Straube A. Hypnic headache: a case presentation including polysomnography. Cephalalgia. 2006;26(1):84–6.
9. Patsouros N, Laloux P, Ossemann M. Hypnic headache: a case report with polysomnography. Acta Neurol Belg. 2004;104(1):37–40.
10. Evers S, Rahmann A, Schwaag S, Lüdermann P, Husstedt IW. Hypnic headache – the first German cases including polysomnography. Cephalalgia. 2003;23(1):20–3.
11. Pinessi L, Rainero I, Cicolin A, Zibetti M, Gentile S, Mutani R. Hypnic headache syndrome: association of the attacks with REM sleep. Cephalalgia. 2003;23(2):150–4.
12. Dodick DW. Polysomnography in hypnic headache syndrome. Headache. 2000;40(9):748–52.
13. Morales F. Síndrome de cefalea hípnica. Revisión. Rev Soc Esp Dolor. 1999;6(5):363–7.
14. Morales-Asín F, Mauri JA, Iñiguez C, Espada F, Mostacero E. The hypnic headache syndrome: report of three new cases. Cephalalgia. 1998;18(3):157–8.
15. Obermann M, Holle D. Hypnic headache. Expert Rev Neurother. 2010;10(9):1391–7.
16. Dexter JD, Weitzman ED. The relationship of nocturnal headaches to sleep stage patterns. Neurology. 1970;20(5):513–8.
17. Dexter JD, Riley TL. Studies in nocturnal migraine. Headache. 1975;15(1):51–62.
18. Silva Néto RP, Almeida KJ. Lithium-responsive headaches. Headache Medicine. 2010;1(1):25–8.

19. Silva-Néto RP, Roesler CP, Raffaelli E Jr. Nocturnal headache, nightmares and lithium. Migrâneas Cefaleias. 2008;11(1):14–6.
20. Martins IP, Gouveia RG. Hypnic headache and travel across time zones: a case report. Cephalalgia. 2001;21(9):928–31.
21. Raskin NH. The hypnic headache syndrome. Headache. 1988;28(8):534–6.
22. Kocasoy-Orhan E, Kayrak-Ertas N, Orhan KS, Ertas M. Hypnic headache syndrome: excessive periodic limb movements in polysomnography. Agri. 2004;16(4):28–30.
23. Dodick DW, Eross EJ, Parish JM, Silber M. Clinical, anatomical, and physiologic relationship between sleep and headache. Headache. 2003;43(3):282–92.
24. Karlovasitou A, Avdelidi E, Andriopoulou G, Baloyannis S. Transient hypnic headache syndrome in a patient with bipolar disorder after the withdrawal of long-term lithium treatment: a case report. Cephalalgia. 2009;29(4):484–6.
25. Somers VK, Dyken ME, Mark AL, Abboud FM. Sympathetic-nerve activity during sleep in normal subjects. N Engl J Med. 1993;328(5):303–7.
26. Cugini P, Granata M, Strano S, Ferrucci A, Ciavarella GM, Di Palma L, et al. Nocturnal headache-hypertension syndrome: a chronobiologic disorder. Chronobiol Int. 1992;9(4):310–3.
27. Holle D, Naegel S, Obermann M. Hypnic headache. Cephalalgia. 2013;33(16):1349–57.
28. Molina-Arjona JA, Jiménez-Jiménez FJ, Vela-Bueno A, Tallón-Barranco A. Hypnic headache associated with stage 3 slow wave sleep. Headache. 2000;40(9):753–4.
29. Holle D, Naegel S, Krebs S, Gaul C, Gizewski E, Diener HC, et al. Hypothalamic gray matter volume loss in hypnic headache. Ann Neurol. 2011;69(3):533–9.
30. Capuano A, Vollono C, Rubino M, Mei D, Cali C, De Angelis A, et al. Hypnic headache: actigraphic and polysomnographic study of a case. Cephalalgia. 2005;25(6):466–9.
31. Headache Classification Subcommittee of the International Headache Society. The international classification of headache disorders, 3rd edition. Cephalalgia. 2018;38(1):1–211.
32. Loh NK, Dinner DS, Foldvary N, Skobieranda F, Yew WW. Do patients with obstructive sleep apnea wake up with headaches? Arch Intern Med. 1999;159(15):1765–8.
33. Aldrich MS, Chauncey JB. Are morning headaches part of obstructive sleep apnea syndrome? Arch Intern Med. 1990;150(6):1265–7.
34. Relja G, Zorzon M, Locatelli L, Carraro N, Antonello RM, Cazzato G. Hypnic headache: rapid and long-lasting response to prednisone in two new cases. Cephalalgia. 2002;22(2):157–9.
35. Queiroz LP, Coral LC. The hypnic headache syndrome – A case report (abstract). Proceedings of 8th congress of the international headache society, 1997 Jun 10-14; Amsterdam, Germany. Cephalalgia. 1997;17(3):303.
36. Ghiotto N, Sances G, Di Lorenzo G, Trucco M, Loi M, Sandrini G, et al. Report of eight new cases of hypnic headache and mini-review of the literature. Funct Neurol. 2002;17(4):211–9.
37. Pinto CAR, Fragoso YD, Souza Carvalho D, Gabbai AA. Hypnic headache syndrome: clinical aspects of eight patients in Brazil. Cephalalgia. 2002;22(10):824–7.
38. Lisoto C, Mainardi F, Maggioni F, Zanchin G. Episodic hypnic headache? Cephalalgia. 2004;24(8):681–5.
39. Manni R, Sances G, Terzaghi M, Ghiotto N, Nappi G. Hypnic headache: PSG evidence of both REM-and NREM-related attacks. Neurology. 2004;62(8):1411–3.
40. Pinto CAR, Fragoso YD, Souza CD. Síndrome da cefaleia hípnica: estudo polissonográfico de 9 pacientes. Migrâneas e Cefaleias. 2003;6(1):15–6.
41. Pascual J. Other primary headaches. Neurol Clin. 2009;27(2):557–71.
42. Cohen AS, Kaube H. Rare nocturnal headaches. Curr Opin Neurol. 2004;17(3):295–9.
43. Holle D, Naegel S, Obermann M. Pathophysiology of hypnic headache. Cephalalgia. 2014;34(10):806–12.
44. Holle D, Naegel S, Krebs S, Katsarava Z, Diener HC, Gaul C, et al. Clinical characteristics and therapeutic options in hypnic headache. Cephalalgia. 2010;30(12):1435–42.
45. Gelfand AA, Goasdby PJ. The role of melatonin in the treatment of primary headache disorders. Headache. 2016;56(8):1257–66.
46. Montagna P. Hypothalamus, sleep and headaches. Neurol Sci. 2006;27(2):138–43.

47. Malick A, Strassman RM, Burstein R. Trigeminohypothalamic and reticulohypothalamic tract neurons in the upper cervical spinal cord and caudal medulla of the rat. J Neurophysiol. 2000;84(4):2078–112.
48. Leone M, Lucini V, D'Amico D, Moschiano F, Maltempo C, Fraschini F, et al. Twenty-four hour melatonin and cortisol plasma levels in relation to timing of cluster headache. Cephalalgia. 1995;15(3):224–9.
49. Treiser SL, Cascio CS, O'Donohue TL, Thoa NB, Jacobowitz DM, Kellar KJ. Lithium increases serotonin release and decreases serotonin receptors in the hippocampus. Science. 1981;213(4515):1529–31.
50. Pablos MI, Santaolaya MJ, Agapito MT, Recio JM. Influence of lithium salts on chick pineal gland melatonin secretion. Neurosci Lett. 1994;174(1):55–7.
51. Lewis AJ, Kerenyi NA, Feuer G. Neuropharmacology of pineal secretion. Drug Metabol Drug Interact. 1990;8(3–4):247–312.
52. Chazot G, Claustrat B, Brun J, Zaidan R. \. Pharmacopsychiatry 1987;20:222–223.
53. Boppana SH, Peterson M, Du AL, Kutikuppala LVS, Gabriel RA. Caffeine: what is its role in pain medicine? Cureus. 2022;14(6):25603.
54. Mathew RJ, Wilson WH. Caffeine induced changes in cerebral circulation. Stroke. 1985;16(5):814–7.
55. Sawynok J. Methylxanthines and pain. Handb Exp Pharmacol. 2011;200:311–29.
56. Zylka MJ. Pain-relieving prospects for adenosine receptors and ectonucleotidases. Trends Mol Med. 2011;17(4):188–96.
57. Huang Z-L, Qu W-M, Eguchi N, et al. Adenosine A_{2A}, but not A_1, receptors mediate the arousal effect of caffeine. Nat Neurosci. 2005;8(7):858–9.
58. Sawynok J. Adenosine receptor activation and nociception. Eur J Pharmacol. 1998;347(1):1–11.
59. Holle D, Obermann M. Hypnic headache and caffeine. Expert Rev Neurother. 2012;12(9):1125–32.
60. Evers S, Goadsby P, Jensen R, May A, Pascual J, Sixt G, et al. Treatment of miscellaneous idiopathic headache disorders (group 4 of the IHS classification) – report of an EFNS task force. Eur J Neurol. 2011;18(6):803–12.
61. Summ O, Andreou AP, Akerman S, Goadsby PJ. A potential nitrergic mechanism of action for indomethacin, but not of other COX inhibitors: relevance to indomethacin-sensitive headaches. J Headache Pain. 2010;11(6):477–83.
62. Summ O, Evers S. Mechanism of action of indomethacin in indomethacin-responsive headaches. Curr Pain Headache Rep. 2013;17(4):327.

Chapter 8
Differential Diagnosis

Doctors believe that once the cause of the disease has been found, its cure has been discovered

Cícero (106–43 a.c.)

Introduction

Although ICHD-3 establishes the diagnostic criteria for hypnic headache and does not include another diagnosis that better explains this disorder [1], many other headaches also occur during sleep or upon awakening [2–4]. Therefore, they are called nocturnal headaches and divided into two groups, primary and secondary, as shown in Table 8.1.

The first group includes nocturnal migraine and the following trigeminal-autonomic headaches: cluster headache, paroxysmal hemicrania, short-lasting unilateral neuralgiform headache attacks with cranial autonomic injection and tearing (SUNCT), and hemicrania continua. All of them should be considered in the differential diagnosis of hypnic headache, due to the similarity of some symptoms [5]. In addition, these headaches have a good therapeutic response with lithium carbonate [6].

The second group comprises the majority of nocturnal headaches. Among secondary headaches, there are headaches attributed to several causes, such as subdural hematoma, non-ruptured vascular malformation, giant cell arteritis, communicating hydrocephalus, intracranial neoplasia, post-ictal nocturnal headache, medication-overuse headache, sleep apnea headache, nocturnal arterial hypertension, and pheochromocytoma [3, 6–9].

Hypnic headache is classified as primary headache. Therefore, it is not attributed to any neurological disorder listed in the group of secondary headaches, it does not have an etiological agent and the patient's neurological examination does not reveal any abnormality [1].

R. Silva-Néto, D. Holle-Lee, *Hypnic Headache*,
https://doi.org/10.1007/978-3-031-32263-1_8

Table 8.1 Classification of nocturnal headaches

ICHD-3 code	Classification
Primary	
1.1	Nocturnal migraine
3.1	Cluster headache
3.2	Paroxysmal hemicranias
3.3	SUNCT and SUNA syndrome
3.4	Hemicrania continua
4.9	Hypnic headache
Secondary	
5.2	Persistent headache attributed to traumatic injury to the head
6.3	Headache attributed to unruptured vascular malformation
6.4.1	Headache attributed to giant cell arteritis
7.1.4	Headache attributed to intracranial hypertension secondary to hydrocephalus
7.4	Headache attributed to intracranial neoplasia
7.6.2	Post-ictal nocturnal headache
8.2	Medication-overuse headache
10.1.4	Sleep apnoea headache
10.3	Headache attributed to arterial hypertension
10.3.1	Headache attributed to phaeochromocytoma
10.7	Headache attributed to other disorder of homoeostasis (hypoglycemia)
12	Headache attributed to psychiatric disorder

Source: Silva-Néto. Cefaleia hípnica: Dores que vem pelo sono. Nova Aliança: Teresina, 2019

Despite this, it is pertinent to make a differential diagnosis with all forms of headache that have a night rhythm. Obviously, the clinical history is fundamental for this diagnosis and the investigation with complementary exams must be planned according to the evidence of the case [9].

Although prevalence decreases with age, headache remains a common neurological complaint among elderly populations. In this age group, secondary headaches are more frequently present, especially when the onset is recent. Migraine and tension-type headaches are rarely new onset in this age group and should be a diagnosis of exclusion [10]. Older adults are about 12 times more likely to have serious underlying causes and often have different symptom presentations compared to younger adults [11].

In hypnic headache, the onset of pain occurs after 50 years of age in 91% of patients [12]. Therefore, when an elderly person complains of nocturnal headache, even fulfilling the diagnostic criteria for hypnic headache, complementary exams should be requested. This investigation includes neuroimaging tests (tomography, magnetic resonance, or angioresonance), polysomnography, and laboratory tests.

In search of a diagnostic accuracy, eventually, other tests are performed, among them, electroencephalogram (EEG) and evoked potentials [8, 13–17], transcranial

Doppler [16–18], routine laboratory tests, including blood count, erythrocyte sedimentation rate and biochemistry [8, 16–23], and CSF examination.

Commonly, in this age group, neuroimaging exams show some intracranial nonspecific abnormalities, such as leukoaraiosis, encephalomalacia, old infarcts, or mild cerebral atrophy [8, 17], but these changes should not be considered as the cause of hypnic headache.

Primary Headaches

Nocturnal Migraine In migraine patients, particularly without aura, headache attacks can occur at any time of the day, including during the night, after sleep onset, or when waking up [24]. In addition to nocturnal headache attacks, migraine patients often have parasomnias, including nocturnal enuresis, sleepwalking, and nightmares.

Although sleep is an improvement factor for migraine, changes in the specific routine of individual sleep, such as an increase or decrease in the amount of sleep and unaccustomed dreams, are the most frequent triggers of headache attacks. Usually, nocturnal headache attacks occur during the central part of sleep, as well as during short daily dreams.

Nocturnal migraine has not yet been sufficiently validated by scientific studies. However, the experts' experience suggests the existence of a primary headache that arises during sleep or upon awakening and fulfills diagnostic criteria for migraine without aura and not for other primary headaches [25–27]. Additional scientific evidence are still required for it to be formally accepted and included in the International Classification of Headaches [25, 27].

According to the Brazilian neurologist Edgard Raffaelli Júnior (1930–2006), as well as menstrual headache, nocturnal migraine does not respond to the usual prophylactic treatments for migraine, suggesting the existence of at least three different neurotransmitter systems [25].

According to ICHD-3, migraine headache is associated with nausea and/or vomiting, photophobia, and phonophobia [1]. However, several studies have shown that headache is also associated with osmophobia [28–30]. In addition to these symptoms, some patients may have parasympathetic autonomic manifestations, including tearing, conjunctival hyperemia, nasal congestion, rhinorrhea, sweating of the face and forehead, miosis, ptosis, and edema of the eyelid [31].

Due to the use of lithium in cyclic evolution pathologies, Raffaelli started to test it in nocturnal migraine. These patients had an absolute therapeutic response to lithium carbonate, at a dose of 300–600 mg/day, in a single dose at night, similar to the treatment of hypnic headache [25, 32].

Cluster Headache Cluster headache is part of the trigeminal autonomic cephalalgias group and has certain peculiarities, such as, for example, excruciating pain, short-term attacks, evident circadian rhythm, periodicity, and autonomic disorders. Usually, the age of onset is 20–40 years. For unknown reasons, men are afflicted three times more often than women [33].

Headache is strictly unilateral, orbital, supraorbital, and temporal or any combination of these sites, but it can spread to other regions. Its intensity varies from severe to very severe, becoming unbearable in the worst attacks. Headache attacks last from 15 to 180 minutes, if left untreated, and a frequency of once every 2 days, up to eight times a day [1].

At least one of the following autonomic manifestations is present ipsilateral to the headache: conjunctival hyperemia, watery eyes, nasal congestion, rhinorrhea, frontal and facial sweating, miosis, ptosis, and edema of the eyelid. Usually, during headache attacks, the patient is unable to lie down and presents restlessness or agitation [1].

Some details not described in ICHD-3 [1] are observed in clinical practice, such as the time when headache attacks occur. A circadian rhythm is observed in 80%–85% of cases. Nocturnal attacks are the most frequent. Approximately, 50%–60% of them occur 90 minutes after the patient falls asleep. Usually, sporadic cases occur during REM sleep, while chronic ones are triggered in all phases of sleep [34].

Paroxysmal Hemicrania Paroxysmal hemicrania is also a trigeminal autonomic cephalalgia and is characterized by being strictly unilateral, associated with autonomic symptoms and/or signs and responsive to indomethacin. It predominates in females [35]. It was first described in 1976 by the Norwegian neurologist Ottar Sjaastad (1928–2022) [25].

Headache, which also manifests at night, is severe, strictly unilateral and located in the orbital, supraorbital, and temporal regions or any combination of these sites. Headache attacks last from 2 to 30 mins, if left untreated, and more than five times a day, for more than half the time [1].

At least one of the following autonomic manifestations is present ipsilateral to the headache: conjunctival hyperemia, watery eyes, nasal congestion, rhinorrhea, eyelid edema, frontal and facial sweating, frontal and facial flushing, feeling of fullness in the ear, miosis, and ptosis [36–38].

SUNCT and SUNA These two syndromes of the trigeminal autonomic cephalalgias group are neuralgiform headaches, strictly unilateral and of very short duration. They are rare, with a clear predominance in males. The term SUNCT means "Short-lasting Unilateral Neuralgiform headache attacks with Conjunctival injection and Tearing"; e SUNA, "Short-lasting Unilateral Neuralgiform headache attacks with Conjunctival injection and Tearing." [1]

Headache is severe, stabbing, strictly unilateral, located in the orbital, supraorbital, temporal, and/or other trigeminal regions, lasting from 1 to 600 seconds, but which is repeated from 3 to 200 times a day [1].

On the same side of pain, at least one of the following parasympathetic cranial symptoms and/or autonomic signs are present: conjunctival hyperemia, tearing, nasal congestion, rhinorrhea, eyelid edema, frontal and facial flushing, feeling of fullness in the ear, miosis, and ptosis. At SUNCT, conjunctival hyperemia and tearing must be present; and at SUNA, only one or none of these two autonomic signals [1].

Hemicrania Continua This headache is characterized by being persistent, strictly unilateral, associated with autonomic symptoms and/or signs, and responsive to indomethacin. It was first described in 1983 by the Norwegian neurologist Ottar Sjaastad (1928–2022) [25].

Headache, which also manifests at night, is of moderate-to-severe intensity, strictly unilateral, without changing sides, in the orbital, supraorbital, temporal regions or any combination of these sites. Pain is continuous if left untreated [1].

At least one of the following parasympathetic autonomic manifestations is present ipsilateral to the headache: conjunctival hyperemia, watery eyes, nasal congestion, rhinorrhea, eyelid edema, frontal and facial sweating, frontal and facial flushing, feeling of fullness in the ear, mycosis, and palpebral ptosis. Usually, during headache attacks, the patient has a feeling of restlessness or agitation, or aggravation of pain by movement [1, 39, 40].

Secondary Headaches

Other headaches occur during sleep, mimicking hypnic headache, but are secondary to other pathologies. Commonly, they are related to the appearance of intracranial lesion or to metabolic disorder demonstrable by appropriate investigation. Headache disappears after removing the cause. In these situations, hypnic headache is called secondary and must be distinguished from the idiopathic form in which there is no secondary cause. These headaches are described in ICHD-3 groups 5–12 [1].

Many cases diagnosed as secondary hypnic headache have already been reported. In these patients, there was another disease that manifested with headache mimicking the hypnic headache. After treating the underlying disease, the hypnic headache disappeared in all patients. Here, we will present secondary hypnic headaches that have already been described in the literature.

Hypnic headache can be secondary to many causes and the main ones are listed below. They can be attributed to traumatic injury to the head, ischemic stroke, non-traumatic subarachnoid hemorrhage, unruptured vascular malformation, arteritis, intracranial hypertension secondary to hydrocephalus, intracranial neoplasia, epileptic seizure (post-ictal headache), use of or exposure to a substance, medication-overuse, disorder of homeostasis (sleep apnea, arterial hypertension, phaeochromocytoma, and hypoglycemia), and psychiatric disorder (depression).

Persistent Headache Attributed to Traumatic Injury to the Head Chronic subdural hematoma is a common diagnosis with a tendency to occur among the elderly. In most cases, it is considered a complication of traumatic brain injury, which causes bleeding by laceration of veins in the subdural space. Elderly people may also develop subdural hematomas as a result of using anti-platelets and anticoagulants. There is a predominance in men (2: 1) [41, 42].

The prevalence of headache in patients with chronic subdural hematoma ranges from 22.6% to 59.5% [41, 43]. It usually starts at night or upon waking and gets worse in the morning [44]. Other signs and symptoms are present, such as altered level of consciousness, impaired gait, hemiparesis, dizziness, aphasia, nausea, and vomiting [41]. The definitive diagnosis is made through tomography or brain resonance [45].

Headache Attributed to Ischemic Stroke A case of hypnic headache secondary to pontine ischemic injury has been described. In this report, a 71-year-old man with a history of hypertension and diabetes mellitus developed right hemiparesis, dysarthria following vertigo, and sudden-onset disequilibrium. Two weeks later, he started having nocturnal headache attacks that started 2–3 h after he fell asleep. A brain MRI was performed which showed an ischemic lesion located in the ventrolateral portion of the midrostral upper pons. This topographic localization corresponds to the pontine reticular formation, where the neural network generating REM sleep is supposed to be located [46].

Acute Headache Attributed to Nontraumatic Subarachnoid Hemorrhage Patients with subarachnoid hemorrhage due to a ruptured aneurysm may experience nocturnal headaches. Recently, a case of hypnic headache that occurred after subarachnoid hemorrhage and clipping and coiling of the distal left internal carotid artery aneurysm was described [47].

Headache Attributed to Unruptured Vascular Malformation Several arterial vascular malformations, such as dolicoectasis, a dilation and elongation of intracranial arteries or veins [48–50] can manifest, clinically, with severe nocturnal headaches and are associated with nausea and/or vomiting. These malformations are evidenced by neuroimaging exams.

Headache Attributed to Giant Cell Arteritis Headache is the most common, but often the only symptom of giant cell arteritis (GCA). It is characterized by being severe, pulsating, continuous, or paroxysmal and located in the region of the temporal arteries, uni or bilateral. It appears gradually at any time of the day, but it usually gets worse at night [9, 51].

The temporal artery is extremely painful on palpation, swollen, and with decreased pulsatility. In addition, the patient may evolve with decreased visual acuity due to impairment of the ciliary, ophthalmic, and central retinal arteries, with blindness occurring in 5%–15% of patients [51–54].

Similar to hypnic headache, GCA is closely linked to the patient's age. It usually starts after the age of 50 years, with a peak incidence between the seventh and eighth decades of life. Its occurrence before the age of 40 years is unusual. Women are affected three times more than men.

Other manifestations of the disease, such as mandibular claudication, nonspecific myalgias, and stiffness of the neck and muscles of the scapular and pelvic girdles, may occur, even after specific treatment has started. Systemic symptoms such as fever, discouragement, fatigue, anorexia, and weight loss occur in 30%–60% of patients and, in some cases, maybe the only symptoms.

Laboratory tests used in the investigation of GCA show that erythrocyte sedimentation rate (ESR) is high in 80% of the patients, conferring a low specificity, but which makes it possible to think about this diagnosis. C-reactive protein is also elevated and when combined with an increase in ESR it gives a greater specificity (97%) in the diagnosis.

Temporal artery biopsy is still the gold standard for the diagnosis of GCA, but it has relatively low sensitivity, around 30%–40%. This sensitivity is increased when the biopsy is performed within 7 days of starting the corticoid and the sample size is greater than 10 mm.

Color duplex-scan ultrasonography visualizes thickening of the temporal artery, in the shape of a halo, with 40% sensitivity and 81% specificity in the diagnosis of GCA. In addition, it is useful in choosing the location of the arterial biopsy. Thus, it is concluded that the presence of a halo sign can prevent the performance of biopsy in cases of high suspicion of GCA and in which there are contraindications for this procedure. High-resolution, contrast-enhanced MRI of the temporal arteries may show inflammation of the arterial walls.

In the presence of a patient who meets diagnostic criteria for hypnic headache, but has an elevated erythrocyte sedimentation rate (ESR), a temporal artery biopsy should be performed [54].

Headache Attributed to Intracranial Hypertension Secondary to Hydrocephalus Headache is the main symptom of intracranial hypertension secondary to hydrocephalus [55]. It is characterized by daily occurrence, especially on waking, frontal, orbital or retro-orbital location, and pressure character.

Usually, the patient gets relief during the day, after getting up, when there is an improvement in venous return and a production of $paCO_2$, but it gets worse with physical activity and/or maneuvers that increase intracranial pressure, such as coughing or physical exertion. It remits with the resolution given hydrocephalus [9].

Other symptoms and / or clinical signs of intracranial hypertension accompany headache, such as nausea and / or vomiting, papilledema, widening of the blind spot, and progressive loss of visual acuity [56]. Occasionally, focal neurological signs are observed, such as motor deficits, ataxia, paralysis of cranial nerves, especially the abducent nerve, decreased level of consciousness, and seizures [57].

Hydrocephalus is diagnosed when the CSF pressure is greater than 250 mmH_2O, in a measure performed by lumbar puncture, in lateral decubitus and without sedative drugs; or by epidural or intraventricular monitoring [1].

Headache Attributed to Intracranial Neoplasia Headache resulting from an intracranial neoplasia can present itself in a similar way to primary headaches, fulfilling the diagnostic criteria for migraine or tension-type headache. This headache is characterized by being intermittent with onset at night or on waking, moderate intensity and associated with vomiting [58–60].

Therefore, headaches that awaken the patient always raise the suspicion of high intracranial pressure. The exclusion of a brain tumor is mandatory whenever headache is associated with vomiting and papilledema [2].

Most often, headache is associated with primary tumors that are located below the tentacle of the cerebellum. Headache lateralization is important, especially in patients with supracentral lesions who do not have increased intracranial pressure [59]. Cases secondary to posterior fossa tumors [60–62], non-secretory pituitary adenoma [63], growth hormone-secreting pituitary adenoma [64], acoustic neuroma [65] have been described.

Post-Ictal Nocturnal Headache Epileptic seizures are strongly influenced by the sleep-wake cycle and, in many patients, they occur, predominantly or exclusively, during sleep [2, 66, 67]. More than 40% of patients with frontotemporal lobe epilepsy and up to 60% of those with occipital lobe epilepsy have post-ictal headache [1, 68], · which are often a diagnostic dilemma.

In this situation, it is necessary to know the characteristics that distinguish epileptic seizures from other paroxysmal nocturnal events [67]. If within 3 h after a partial or generalized nocturnal epileptic seizure, the patient developed headache lasting up to 72 h, the diagnosis of post-ictal headache is confirmed [1].

Attributed to a Substance or Its Withdrawal The headache most often attributed to substance use is medication overuse headache (MOH). Patients who have primary headaches, such as migraine, usually self-medicate and develop secondary headache from overuse of medications. This headache can manifest at night and for 15 or more days per month [2, 69].

MOH shows clinical improvement when there is a reduction in the use of painkillers, but does not respond to drugs, usually used in the treatment of hypnic headache [69].

Some headaches are associated with withdrawal from a substance. A case report describes an 84-year-old woman who had her angiotensin-converting enzyme (ACE) inhibitor abruptly stopped. She immediately developed a headache that woke her up at 3 am every night. After restarting the ACE inhibitor, her headache was completely gone [70].

Sleep Apnea Headache Headache is a recognized symptom of sleep apnea syndrome. It is characterized by occurring upon awakening, usually bilateral, having a pressure character, moderate intensity, and lasting less than 4 h [9]. It is not accompanied by nausea, photophobia, or phonophobia. Headache usually remites after treatment of sleep apnea with continuous positive airway pressure (CPAP) [1].

The definitive diagnosis of this disorder is made through polysomnography at night, which should show an apnea/hypopnea index ≥5 [71].

Sleep apnea manifests with nocturnal or morning headache [72, 73], but its presence does not necessarily exclude the diagnosis of hypnic headache [1]. In a series of cases with polysomnography in hypnic headache, sleep apnea syndrome was not found, despite these two conditions coexisting [13, 16, 74].

Headache Attributed to Arterial Hypertension Hypnic headache must also be distinguished from nocturnal arterial hypertension, another possible chronobiological disorder [74]. Patients under inadequate treatment for hypertension may have recurrent episodes of increased blood pressure during sleep, causing awakening followed by headache. This headache disappears after antihypertensive therapy [75, 76].

There are reports of two cases of patients with arterial hypertension who had headache during sleep associated with increased blood pressure levels. In both, pain was relieved by antihypertensive therapy. One of them underwent ambulatory blood pressure monitoring (ABPM) which confirmed nocturnal arterial hypertension. From these reports, it is concluded that it is important to include ABPM to assess complaints of nocturnal headache, especially in the elderly, in whom essential hypertension is a frequent comorbidity [17, 76].

Headache Attributed to Phaeochromocytoma Pheochromocytoma is a catecholamine-producing neuroendocrine tumor and usually benign. In 90% of patients, it is located in the adrenal glands, but it can originate in paraganglia of the bifurcation of the iliac arteries and bladder, chest, and brain [77]. It is considered a rare cause of secondary hypertension, with prevalence ranging from 0.1% to 0.6% [78]. It occurs at any age, with equal gender distribution [79].

The classic symptoms of pheochromocytoma are headache, high blood pressure, tachycardia, and nocturnal diaphoresis, but other symptoms may be present, including abdominal pain, tremors, and constipation [77, 79].

Usually, the headache is located in the frontal region, bilaterally, with temporal irradiation or, more rarely, occipital. It lasts from a few minutes to hours and has a frequency of one to three episodes per day. In general, it can wake the patient up at night or appear as soon as he wakes up [9].

In diagnostic investigation, the levels of plasma catecholamines, norepinephrine, epinephrine, and dopamine or their urinary metabolites, vanillylmandelic acid, metanephrine, and normetanephrine are measured. Provocative tests with glucagon and suppressive tests with clonidine can also be done. Radiological evaluation should be done when biochemical measurements confirm the diagnosis of catecholamine-secreting tumor. Abdominal magnetic resonance is used, whose sensitivity is 95% [9, 77, 79].

Headache Attributed to Other Disorders of Homeostasis (hypoglycemia) Hypoglycemia is defined when the blood glucose level is below the range considered normal, that is, 60 mg/dl and, commonly, it happens in people who have diabetes. It is classified as mild, moderate, or severe, until reaching the glycemic coma, if not treated in time.

Among the most common causes are diabetes, prolonged fasting, a diet high in hypoglycemic carbohydrates, insulin overdose or oral hypoglycemic agents, post-gastrectomies, insulinomas, hypopituitarism, and Addison's disease [9].

Clinical symptoms of hypoglycemia can be attributable to adrenergic responses (tremor, tachycardia, pallor, sweating, mydriasis, etc.) and brain dysfunction (such as headache, mental confusion, seizures, and coma) [80]. Nocturnal hypoglycemia is quite common, so headache also manifests at night and is usually diffuse in location. Diagnosis can be confirmed by laboratory tests, such as fasting glycemic curve, postprandial and after glucose overload, in addition to tolbutamide tolerance test [9, 81, 82].

There is a case report of a 64-year-old woman presenting headaches exclusively during sleep and fulfilling the diagnostic criteria for hypnic headache, but a 72-hour glucose monitoring showed hypoglycemia episodes related to the onset of headaches. The disappearance of headache attacks after correction of nocturnal hypoglycemia pointed to a cause and effect relationship between hypoglycemia and hypnic headache. The authors hypothesized that insufficient glucose supply in the suprachiasmatic nucleus and hypothalamus could trigger headache attacks in predisposed individuals. These structures have glucose as the main source of energy. Faced with hypoglycemia, they will be unable to function properly [82].

Other Causes Headache secondary to illicit drug withdrawal may occur predominantly at night [9]. Depression is a treatable medical condition that is easily identifiable in clinical evaluation and it can interrupt sleep and cause headache at night or upon awakening [2, 81]. There is a case report of a patient diagnosed with idiopathic cyclic edema who presented with headache upon awakening. After generalized edema, he developed headache that started around 5–6 am and disappeared spontaneously 3–4 h after waking up. After treatment with aminaphtone, which interferes in the capillary permeability, the generalized edema and headache completely disappeared [83]. Nonvascular intracranial disorders such as intracranial hypotension can be a cause of hypnic headache [84].

Primary nocturnal headaches described above should be remembered in the differential diagnosis of hypnic headache, but there is the possibility of coexistence of hypnic headache with other night headaches in the same patient. Associations between hypnic headache and migraine [85] or SUNCT [86] were described.

References

1. Headache Classification Subcommittee of the International Headache Society. The international classification of headache disorders, 3rd edition. Cephalalgia. 2018;38(1):1–211.
2. Larner AJ. Not all morning headaches are due to brain tumours. Pract Neurol. 2009;9(2):80–4.
3. Evans RW, Dodick DW, Schwedt TJ. The headaches that awaken us. Headache. 2006;46(4):678–81.
4. Cohen AS, Kaube H. Rare nocturnal headaches. Curr Opin Neurol. 2004;17(3):295–9.

5. Casucci G. Chronic short-lasting headaches: clinical features and differential diagnosis. Neurol Sci. 2003;24(2):101–7.
6. Silva-Néto RP, Roesler CP, Raffaelli E Jr. Nocturnal headache, nightmares and lithium. Migrâneas Cefaleias. 2008;11(1):14–6.
7. Sandrini G, Tassorelli C, Ghiotto N, Nappi G. Uncommon primary headaches. Curr Opin Neurol. 2006;19(3):299–304.
8. Evers S, Goadsby PJ. Hypnic headache. Pract Neurol. 2005;5(3):144–9.
9. Sanvito WL, Monzillo PH. O livro das cefaleias. São Paulo: Atheneu; 2001.
10. Robblee J, Singh RH. Headache in the older population: causes, diagnoses, and treatments. Curr Pain Headache Rep. 2020;24(7):34.
11. Kaniecki RG, Levin AD. Headache in the elderly. Handb Clin Neurol. 2019;167:511–28.
12. Silva-Néto RP, Sousa-Santos PEM, Peres MFP. Hypnic headache: a review of 348 cases published from 1988 to 2018. J Neurol Sci. 2019;401:103–9.
13. Evers S, Rahmann A, Schwaag S, Lüdermann P, Husstedt IW. Hypnic headache – the first German cases including polysomnography. Cephalalgia. 2003;23(1):20–3.
14. Capo G, Esposito A. Hypnic headache. A new Italian case with a good response to pizotifene and melatonin (abstract). Proceedings of 10th congress of the international headache society, 2001 Jun 29 to Jul 3; New York, EUA. Cephalalgia. 2001;21(4):505–6.
15. Relja G, Zorzon M, Locatelli L, Carraro N, Antonello RM, Cazzato G. Hypnic headache: rapid and long-lasting response to prednisone in two new cases. Cephalalgia. 2002;22(2):157–9.
16. Pinessi L, Rainero I, Cicolin A, Zibetti M, Gentile S, Mutani R. Hypnic headache syndrome: association of the attacks with REM sleep. Cephalalgia. 2003;23(2):150–4.
17. Gil-Gouveia R, Goadsby PJ. Secondary hypnic headache. J Neurol. 2007;254(5):646–54.
18. Centonze V, D'Amico D, Usai S, Causarano V, Bassi A, Bussone G. First Italian case of hypnic headache, with literature review and discussion of nosology. Cephalalgia. 2001;21(1):71–4.
19. Patsouros N, Laloux P, Ossemann M. Hypnic headache: a case report with polysomnography. Acta Neurol Belg. 2004;104(1):37–40.
20. Zanchin G, Lisotto C, Maggioni F. The hypnic headache syndrome: the first description of an Italian case. J Headache Pain. 2000;1(1):60.
21. Ivañez V, Soler R, Barreiro P. Hypnic headache syndrome: a case with good response to indomethacin. Cephalalgia. 1998;18(4):225–6.
22. Morales-Asín F, Mauri JA, Iñiguez C, Espada F, Mostacero E. The hypnic headache syndrome: report of three new cases. Cephalalgia. 1998;18(3):157–8.
23. Gould JD, Silberstein SD. Unilateral hypnic headache: a case study. Neurology. 1997;49(6):1749–51.
24. Alberti A. Headache and sleep. Sleep Med Rev. 2006;10(6):431–7.
25. Silva-Néto R. Cefaleias noturnas. In: Silva-Néto R, editor. Cefaleia – aspectos históricos e tópicos relevantes. Teresina: Halley; 2013. p. 139–44.
26. Dexter JD, Riley TL. Studies in nocturnal migraine. Headache. 1975;15(1):51–62.
27. Dexter JD. Studies in nocturnal migraine. Arch Neurobiol (Madr). 1974;37:281–300.
28. Silva-Néto RP, Peres MFP, Valença MM. Accuracy of osmophobia in the differential diagnosis between migraine and tension-type headache. J Neurol Sci. 2014;339:118–22.
29. De Carlo D, Dal Zotto L, Perissinotto E, Gallo L, Gatta M, Balottin U, et al. Osmophobia in migraine classification - a multicentre study in juvenile patients. Cephalalgia. 2010;30(12):1486–94.
30. Porta-Etessam JP, García-Morales I, Di Capua D, García-Cobos R. A patient with primary sexual headache associated with hypnic headaches. J Headache Pain. 2009;10(2):135.
31. Obermann M, Yoon MS, Dommes P, Kuznetsova J, Maschke M, Weimar C, et al. Prevalence of trigeminal autonomic symptoms in migraine: a population-based study. Cephalalgia. 2007;27(6):504–9.
32. Silva Néto RP, Almeida KJ. Lithium-responsive headaches. Headache Medicine. 2010;1(1):25–8.

33. Cruz S, Lemos C, Monteiro JM. Familial aggregation of cluster headache. Arq Neuropsiquiatr. 2013;71(11):866–70.
34. Pfaffenrath V, Pollman W, Ruther E, Lund R, Hajak G. Onset of nocturnal attacks of chronic cluster headache in relation to sleep stages. Acta Neurol Scand. 1986;73(4):403–7.
35. Vincent MB. Hemicrania continua. Unquestionably a trigeminal autonomic cephalalgia. Headache. 2013;53(5):863–8.
36. Beams JL, Rozen TD. Paroxysmal hemicrania as the clinical presentation of giant cell arteritis. Clin Pract. 2011;1(4):111.
37. Prakash S, Patell R. Paroxysmal hemicrania: an update. Curr Pain Headache Rep. 2014;18(4):407.
38. Prakash S, Belani P, Susvirkar A, Trivedi A, Ahuja S, Patel A. Paroxysmal hemicrania: a retrospective study of a consecutive series of 22 patients and a critical analysis of the diagnostic criteria. J Headache Pain. 2013;14(1):26.
39. Charlson RW, Robbins MS. Hemicrania continua. Curr Neurol Neurosci Rep. 2014;14(3):436.
40. Goasdby PJ. Hemicrania continua-building on experience and clinical science. J Headache Pain. 2014;13(15):9.
41. Yamada SM, Tomita Y, Murakami H, Nakane M, Yamada S, Murakami M, et al. Headache in patients with chronic subdural hematoma: analysis in 1080 patients. Neurosurg Rev. 2018;41(2):549–56.
42. Farhat Neto J, Araujo JL, Ferraz VR, Haddad L, Veiga JC. Chronic subdural hematoma: epidemiological and prognostic analysis of 176 cases. Rev Col Bras Cir. 2015;42(5):283–7.
43. Gelabert-González M, Frieiro-Dantas C, Serramito-García R, Díaz-Cabanas L, Aran-Echabe E, Rico-Cotelo M, et al. Chronic subdural hematoma in young patients. Neurocirugia (Astur). 2013;24(2):63–9.
44. Pereira CU, Santos Junior JA, Santos ANL, Passos RO. Hematoma subdural crônico em adultos jovens. Arq Bras Neurocir. 2015;34:25–9.
45. Traynelis VC. Chronic subdural hematoma in the elderly. Clin Geriatr Med. 1991;7(3):583–98.
46. Moon HS, Chung CS, Hong SB, Kim YB, Chung PW. A case of symptomatic hypnic headache syndrome. Cephalalgia. 2006;26(1):81–3.
47. Aldred MP, Raviskanthan S, Mortensen PW, Lee AG. Hypnic headaches in a patient post coiling and clipping of intracranial aneurysm. J Neuroophthalmol. 2021;42(1):415–6.
48. Fonseca M, Teotónio P, Fonseca AC. An unsuspected cause of hypnic-like headache. J Neurol. 2016;264(2):404–6.
49. Moreira IM, Mendonça T, Monteiro JP, Santos E. Hypnic headache and basilar artery dolichoectasia. Neurologist. 2015;20(6):106–7.
50. Smith AR, Carpenter J, Pergami P. Nocturnal headaches and pulsatile cranial mass: the tip of an iceberg. Pediatr Neurol. 2013;49(5):358–60.
51. Nesher G, Breuer GS. Giant cell arteritis and polymyalgia Rheumatica: 2016 update. Rambam Maimonides Med J. 2016;7(4):e0035.
52. Coffin-Pichonnet S, Bienvenu B, Mouriaxu F. Ophthalmological complications of giant cell arteritis. J Fr Ophtalmol. 2013;36(2):178–83.
53. Figus M, Talarico R, Posarelli C, d'Ascanio A, Elefante E, Bombardieri S. Ocular involvement in giant cell arteritis. Clin Exp Rheumatol. 2013;31(75):96.
54. Lisoto C, Mainardi F, Maggioni F, Zanchin G. Episodic hypnic headache? Cephalalgia. 2004;24(8):681–5.
55. Bouzerar R, Tekaya I, Bouzerar R, Balédent. Dynamics of hydrocephalus: a physical approach. J Biol Phys. 2012;38(2):251–66.
56. Qvarlander S, Lundkvist B, Koskinen LO, Malm J, Eklund A. Pulsatility in CSF dynamics: pathophysiology of idiopathic normal pressure hydrocephalus. J Neurol Neurosurg Psychiatry. 2013;84(7):735–41.
57. García M, Poza J, Santamarta D, Abásolo D, Barrio P, Hornero R. Spectral analysis of intracranial pressure signals recorded during infusion studies in patients with hydrocephalus. Med Eng Phys. 2013;35(10):1490–8.

58. Nelson S, Taylor LP. Headaches in brain tumor patients: primary or secondary? Headache. 2014;54(4):776–85.
59. Suwanwela N, Phanthumchinda K, Kaoropthum S. Headache in brain tumor: a cross-sectional study. Headache. 1994;34(7):435–8.
60. Rossi LN, Vassella F. Headache in children with brain tumors. Childs Nerv Syst. 1989;5(5):307–9.
61. Mullally WJ, Hall KE. Hypnic headache secondary to haemangioblastoma of the cerebellum. Cephalalgia. 2010;30(7):887–9.
62. Peatfield RC, Mendoza ND. Posterior fossa meningioma presenting as hypnic headache. Headache. 2003;43(9):1007–8.
63. Garza I, Oas KH. Symptomatic hypnic headache secondary to a nonfunctioning pituitary macroadenoma. Headache. 2009;49(3):470–2.
64. Valentinis L, Tuniz F, Mucchiut M, Vindigni M, Skrap M, Bergonzi P, et al. Hypnic headache secondary to a growth hormone-secreting pituitary tumour. Cephalalgia. 2008;29(1):82–4.
65. Ceronie B, Green F, Cockerell OC. Acoustic neuroma presenting as a hypnic headache. BMJ Case Rep. 2021;14(3):e235830.
66. Nobili L, Proserpio P, Combi R, Provini F, Plazzi G, Bisulli F, et al. Nocturnal frontal lobe epilepsy. Curr Neurol Neurosci Rep. 2014;14(2):424.
67. Husain AM, Sinha SR. Nocturnal epilepsy in adults. J Clin Neurophysiol. 2011;28(2):141–5.
68. Cianchetti C, Pruna D, Ledda M. Epileptic seizures and headache/migraine: a review of types of association and terminology. Seizure. 2013;22(9):679–85.
69. Baykan B, Ertas M. Hypnic headache associated with medication overuse: case report. Agri. 2008;20(3):40–3.
70. Eccles MJ, Gutowski NJ. Precipitation of long duration hypnic headaches after ACE inhibitor withdrawal. J Neurol. 2007;254(11):1597–8.
71. Alberti A, Mazzotta G, Gallinella E, Sarchielli P. Headache characteristics in obstructive sleep apnea syndrome and insomnia. Acta Neurol Scand. 2005;111(5):309–16.
72. Loh NK, Dinner DS, Foldvary N, Skobieranda F, Yew WW. Do patients with obstructive sleep apnea wake up with headaches? Arch Intern Med. 1999;159(15):1765–8.
73. Aldrich MS, Chauncey JB. Are morning headaches part of obstructive sleep apnea syndrome? Arch Intern Med. 1990;150(6):1265–7.
74. Manni R, Sances G, Terzaghi M, Ghiotto N, Nappi G. Hypnic headache: PSG evidence of both REM-and NREM-related attacks. Neurology. 2004;62(8):1411–3.
75. Cugini P, Granata M, Strano S, Ferrucci A, Ciavarella GM, Di Palma L, et al. Nocturnal headache-hypertension syndrome: a chronobiologic disorder. Chronobiol Int. 1992;9(4):310–3.
76. Silva-Néto RP, Bernardino SN. Ambulatory blood pressure monitoring in patient with hypnic headache: a case study. Headache. 2013;53(7):1157–8.
77. Malachias MVB. Feocromocitoma – diagnóstico e tratamento. Rev Bras Hipertens. 2002;9(2):160–4.
78. Anderson G Jr, Blakeman N, Streeten D. The effect of age on prevalence of secondary forms of hypertension in 4429 consecutively referred patients. J Hypertens. 1994;12(5):609–15.
79. Tsirlin A, Oo Y, Sharma R, Kansara A, Gliwa A, Banerji MA. Pheochromocytoma: a review. Maturitas. 2014;77(3):229–38.
80. Berge LI, Riise T, Fasmer OB, Hundal O, Oedegaard KJ, Midthjell K, et al. Does diabetes have a protective effect on migraine? Epidemiology. 2013;24(1):129–34.
81. Dodick DW, Eross EJ, Parish JM, Silber M. Clinical, anatomical, and physiologic relationship between sleep and headache. Headache. 2003;43(3):282–92.
82. Silva-Néto RP, Soares AA, Peres MFP. Hypnic headache due to hypoglycemia: a case report. Headache. 2019;59(8):1370–3.
83. Godoy JM. Remission of hypnic headache associated with idiopathic cyclic edema with the use of aminaphtone. Open Neurol J. 2010;4:90–1.

84. Freeman WD, Brazis TW, Capobianco DJ, et al. Hypnic headache and intracranial hypotension. In: Proceedings of 46th Annual Scientific Meeting American Headache Society, 2004 Jun 10–13; Vancouver, British Columbia. Headache. 2004;44(5):498.
85. Ruiz M, Mulero P, Pedraza MI, de la Cruz C, Rodríguez C, Muñoz I, et al. From wakefulness to sleep: migraine and hypnic headache association in a series of 23 patients. Headache. 2015;55(1):167–73.
86. Fantini J, Granato A, Zorzon M, Manganotti P. Case report: coexistence of SUNCT and hypnic headache in the same patient. Headache. 2016;56(9):1503–6.

Chapter 9
Treatment

Science finds remedies faster than answers

Jean Rostand (1894–1977)

Introduction

Treatment and management of hypnic headache is a challenging task and requires a thorough evaluation. They must be understood in two ways. First, the abortive headache attacks, in which drugs are administered as soon as the pain appears; and second, the prophylactic, in order to prevent the recurrence of these headache attacks.

Currently, successful treatment, both acute and prophylactic, is based on some series or case reports. However, no randomized clinical trial has been conducted. Thus, treatment recommendations are based on observational studies and need further validation [1].

Only the efficacy of the medications should not be considered, but also their adverse effects, since most patients are elderly and have some comorbidities. Therapeutic options and responses to treatment are shown in Tables 9.1, 9.2, and 9.3.

R. Silva-Néto, D. Holle-Lee, *Hypnic Headache*,
https://doi.org/10.1007/978-3-031-32263-1_9

Table 9.1 Acute treatment used for hypnic headache attacks

Treatment	n	Efficacy			Response rate
		None	Partial (A)	Good (B)	(A + B/n, %)
Caffeine [8, 12, 14–18]	28	6	3	19	78.6
Caffeine-containing analgesics [6, 8, 15, 16, 19, 20]	15	4	2	9	73.3
Acetylsalicylic acid [6, 10, 19, 21–23]	7	3	3	1	57.1
Hypnotics and sedatives [24–26]	3	1	0	2	66.7
Ergotamine and derivatives [10, 17, 27, 28]	4	3	1	0	25.0
Opiates [14, 15, 28, 29]	4	3	0	1	25.0
Oxygen inhalation [4, 15, 21, 27, 29, 30]	9	7	0	2	22.2
Dipyron or acetaminophen [3, 5, 9, 15, 29, 31–34]	21	17	2	2	19.0
Triptans [3, 15, 19, 21, 27, 28, 30, 35, 36]	38	31	2	5	18.4
NSAIDs [3, 6, 9, 15, 18, 25, 27, 28, 30, 33–35, 37, 38]	54	47	4	3	13.0

NSAIDs: non-steroidal anti-inflammatory drugs
Source: Silva-Néto RP, Sousa-Santos PEM, Peres MFP. Hypnic headache: A review of 348 cases published from 1988 to 2018. J Neurol Sci 2019;401:103-9

Table 9.2 Medications used in the prophylactic treatment for hypnic headache

Treatment	n	Efficacy			Response rate
		None	Partial (A)	Good (B)	(A + B/n, %)
Lithium [3, 7, 8, 10–15, 18, 24, 27, 28, 33, 35–57]	129	35	9	85	72.9
Caffeine [3, 7, 10, 12, 15, 19, 21, 28, 33–35, 38, 58]	69	32	17	20	53.6
Indomethacin [3, 10, 12, 14, 15, 17, 18, 22, 25, 27–30, 34–38, 40, 43, 46, 48, 55, 57, 59–65]	71	35	4	32	50.7
Melatonin [3, 10, 14, 15, 27, 34, 35, 38, 66]	26	13	2	11	50.0
Topiramate [3, 14, 15, 35, 53, 57, 62, 67]	31	18	6	7	41.9
Flunarizine [8, 10, 14, 21, 29, 35, 36, 38, 44, 49, 53, 54, 63, 64, 66, 68, 69]	52	31	1	20	40.4
Beta-adrenergic blockers [3, 8, 10, 12, 30, 36–38, 41, 49, 70–72]	18	13	1	4	27.8
Tricyclic antidepressants [3, 6, 8, 15, 19, 21, 27, 28, 30, 32, 35–37, 41, 48, 49, 57, 70, 73, 74]	50	39	2	9	22.0
Gabapentin [3, 28, 34, 37, 38, 63]	9	4	1	4	55.5
Prednisone [9, 12, 18, 27, 28, 38]	7	4	1	2	42.9
Verapamil [3, 10, 21, 27, 28, 36, 38, 49]	11	8	0	3	27.3
Pizotifene [10, 36–38, 49]	5	4	0	1	20.0

Table 9.2 (continued)

Treatment	n	Efficacy			Response rate (A + B/n, %)
		None	Partial (A)	Good (B)	
SSRIs [3, 24, 27, 30, 37, 40, 48]	9	9	0	0	0.0
Lamotrigine [5, 32]	3	0	0	3	100.0
Oxetorone [16]	8	0	8	0	100.0
Valproic acid/sodium divalproate [29, 30, 36, 49]	5	5	0	0	0.0

SSRIs selective serotonin reuptake inhibitors
Source: Silva-Néto RP, Sousa-Santos PEM, Peres MFP. Hypnic headache: A review of 348 cases published from 1988 to 2018. J Neurol Sci 2019;401:103-9

Table 9.3 Efficacy of prophylactics for hypnic headache

Probably effective (WILL HAPPEN)	Possibly effective (IT MAY HAPPEN)	Probably ineffective (WILL NOT HAPPEN)	New options
Lithium Caffeine Indomethacin Melatonin	Topiramate Lamotrigine Gabapentin Flunarizine	Beta-adrenergic blockers Tricyclic antidepressants SSRIs Verapamil Pizotifene Valproic acid Sodium valproate	Botulinic toxin Nerve stimulation Nerve block

SSRIs: selective serotonin reuptake inhibitors
Source: Silva-Néto RP, Sousa-Santos PEM, Peres MFP. Hypnic headache: A review of 348 cases published from 1988 to 2018. J Neurol Sci 2019;401:103-9

Abortive Treatment

Most headache attacks are of moderate intensity, with spontaneous remission within a few hours and do not need acute treatment. Only a third of patients have severe headache and need abortive treatment [2].

In an attempt to obtain pain relief, even if incomplete, patients develop attitudes that do not always result in improvement. Some motor behaviors during each headache episode, mainly sitting up in bed or in an armchair, getting up, and walking showed some benefit [3–12]. It is believed that the improvement in pain when standing up and walking around the room may be related to an increase in cerebral blood flow that varies with posture and physical activity, altering vascular tone [13].

In order to improve their pain, some patients use other non-pharmacological measures, such as using an ice pack or heat on the head, sleeping with several pillows or even eating, reading, and watching television [5, 10, 12]. There is no information as to whether diet or lifestyle changes influence the clinical course of the disease.

In more than 80% of patients, the duration of pain is less than 2 hours, so it is difficult to administer an abortion treatment [2]. Despite this difficulty, some drugs have been tested, still in a few patients, and the results are not encouraging. Table 9.1 summarized the reported efficacy of different acute treatments, classified according to the statements of the respective authors.

Caffeine, isolated or associated with analgesics, was the treatment that showed the best efficacy, with a response rate greater than 70% [12, 14–16, 18], although its underlying pharmacological mechanisms for hypnic headache are still not very clear. However, most patients did not want to try this treatment option because they were afraid of insomnia.

For this good response during headache attacks that awaken the patient, it is recommended to ingest caffeine in the form of a cup of coffee, caffeine capsules, or painkillers containing caffeine. However, it is good to remember that daily intake of painkillers can lead to the onset of medication-overuse headache.

Despite the good response rate, hypnotics and sedatives were used in a few patients [24–26]. Thus, acetylsalicylic acid proved to be the second most useful option for acute treatment, with a response rate equal to 57.1% [19, 21, 23]. Other non-steroidal anti-inflammatory drugs have also been tested, but without efficacya [3, 6, 9, 15, 18, 25, 27, 28, 30, 33–35, 37, 38]. Ergotamine, common analgesics, and triptans were tried. Their response rates were 25%, 19%, and 18.4%, respectively.

Inhalation of 100% oxygen, which works very well in cluster headache, was tested in nine patients with hypnic headache, but relieved headache in only two of them, giving a response rate equal to 22%.

Prophylactic Treatment

In clinical practice, the treatment of hypnic headache is focused on the prophylactic approach with the continuous use of drugs, before going to sleep, to prevent the occurrence of headache attacks during sleep. Observation of reported cases over the past 34 years shows that drug treatment is undoubtedly effective. However, there is a description of non-pharmacological preventive treatment, consisting of an alarm clock to turn off after 4 hours of sleep and which was often able to prevent headache attacks [38]. There is also a report in which the episodes resolved spontaneously, without the administration of any treatment [39].

Numerous drugs are part of the therapeutic arsenal tested in the prophylaxis of hypnic headache, among them: lithium carbonate, caffeine, indomethacin, calcium channel blockers, beta-adrenergic blockers, antidepressants (tricyclic and SSRIs), anticonvulsants, serotonergic antagonists, melatonin, corticosteroids, and miscellaneous. Of all these drugs, only three showed good reasons for successful versus unsuccessful attempts in more than 78% (269/345) of patients. The following should be considered as effective preventive treatment options: lithium carbonate, caffeine, and indomethacin (Table 9.2).

In assessing the therapeutic response, only the drugs tested in at least three patients are shown in Table 9.2. Effectiveness is classified according to the statements of the respective authors. While there is a lack of good quality clinical data for the management of hypnic headache, the following medications have shown benefit in their management.

Lithium Lithium (from Greek *lithos*, stone) is a chemical element with symbol Li, discovered by Johan August Arfwedson (1792–1841) in 1817, from minerals from a petalite mine on the island of Utö, Sweden. It received this name because it was discovered in a mineral, although it was later found in the ashes of plants. In addition to petalite, lithium can be extracted from other minerals, such as, for example, lepidolite, spodumene, and amblygonite [75, 76].

In nature, lithium is found in various forms, such as salts, chloride, bromide, stearate, and hydroxide, but only lithium salts are used in medicine, particularly lithium carbonate (Li_2CO_3) [75, 76].

Initially, lithium carbonate was classified as an anti-psychotic and today, due to its mood-regulating effects, it is used as an anti-manic and, secondarily, an antidepressant. Among its mechanisms of action, prolactin inhibition and prostaglandin synthesis are known, in addition to acting on monoamines, cAMP, platelets, and sleep [75, 76].

It is not yet well understood how lithium carbonate acts in hypnic headache, but some studies have shown its effectiveness in several chronobiological disorders with cyclical evolution, such as bipolar disorder, cluster headache, and nocturnal migraine, besides being the drug of choice for treat nightmares [39, 75, 76].

It is known that lithium leads to an increase in the serum level of melatonin [77–79], which may be important in the pathophysiology of hypnic headache. In addition, lithium causes negative regulation of serotonergic receptors and increased serotonin release [80], suggesting an involvement of the metabolism of this neurotransmitter in hypnic headache, which may also explain the good response to triptans in some cases [15]. Possibly, lithium stabilizes and increases serotonergic transmission at the central nervous system (CNS) level, particularly in the hypothalamus.

Raskin, in 1988, showed the first evidence of the effectiveness of lithium in the treatment of hypnic headache [39]. Subsequently, several other studies were published, confirming their findings. To date, lithium is the most used drug in the prophylactic treatment of hypnic headache, with a response rate of 72.9% (Table 9.1) and suggested as the first choice. Several studies have shown better efficacy in the daily dose of 300–1200 mg, once a day, administered at bedtime to maintain a serum level of 0.5–1.0 mmol/L. [40, 70, 71, 81, 82]

Evidence of the therapeutic response of this drug has been demonstrated in several studies [8, 11, 13, 18, 24, 33, 40, 41, 44, 45, 47–50, 54, 56, 59, 70]. In all studies, after 2 weeks of treatment, when there was an improvement in the frequency and intensity of headache attacks, lithium was replaced by placebo and the headache returned within 1–5 days. Resumption of lithium again resulted in improvement of the headache, however, when treatment was stopped, the headache reappeared in most patients.

Although previous studies have shown a rapid response to lithium, recent studies suggest a slow onset of action. In some patients, lithium can show its full beneficial effects as an antidepressant and mood stabilizer within 2 months. Therefore, it is recommended to give this drug a reasonable time to establish its therapeutic effect in patients with hypnic headache [2].

It is worth mentioning that hypnic headache affects, in most cases, patients over 50 years of age. In this age group, the coexistence of arterial hypertension is common and commonly treated with diuretics. However, lithium should not be used concomitantly with a low sodium diet or with diuretics that induce sodium loss, since sodium depletion causes intracellular lithium retention [12, 75].

Although lithium carbonate is described as an effective treatment, sometimes its adverse effects contraindicate its prescription and require interruption of treatment, even at doses below 600 mg daily. Among these effects, it is commonly reported the appearance of hand tremors or worsening of pre-existing tremors. More rarely, extrapyramidal effects, drowsiness, vertigo, decreased thyroid hormones, disturbances of consciousness (confused night state with agitation), mild renal dysfunction, electrocardiographic changes, psoriasis, and worsening of headache attacks appear [12, 15, 36, 39, 42, 46, 54, 55, 57].

This lithium intolerance must be taken into account [83]. Perhaps because of fear of adverse effects, some patients refuse to use lithium as a treatment for hypnic headache [19, 42].

Caffeine Caffeine is an alkaloid with the chemical structure "3,7-dihydro-1,3,7-trimethyl-1H-purine-2,6-dione." It is an alkaloid belonging to the group of methylxanthines, together with theobromine and theophylline. The effects of caffeine were first recognized in 850 by a "goat herder" named "Khaldi" in southern Abyssinia (currently Ethiopia). However, a German scientist named Friedlieb Ferdinand Runge, in 1819, extracted it for the first time [84].

Pharmacologically, caffeine is a competitive antagonist of adenosine receptors (A_1, A_{2A}, and A_{2B}). This, in turn, reduces cortical hyperexcitability and causes cerebral vasodilation. Therefore, caffeine becomes a potent cerebral vasoconstrictor by blocking the action of adenosine [85]. Furthermore, caffeine inhibits phosphodiesterase at a central level. Thus, there is no degradation of cyclic AMP, which acts as a second messenger in serotonergic receptors.

It is found in caffeinated beverages, such as coffee, black tea, chocolate, cola-type soft drinks, and guarana, and in combination with common pain relievers, ergot derivatives, and non-steroidal anti-inflammatory drugs [86].

Caffeine when ingested, both as a caffeinated drink (1–2 cups), and in pill form (50–300 mg), was an effective treatment for hypnic headache in several reported cases, with a response rate of 53.6% (Table 9.2). This drug is well accepted for not having serious adverse effects [71]. It is well tolerated in the elderly population and, surprisingly, does not interfere with sleep. However, most patients do not want to try this treatment option because they are afraid of going without sleep. Therefore, caffeine is often used as a first-line treatment for this headache [82].

Some important factors should be considered before starting caffeine use, such as dependence and risk of withdrawal headache [2]. Caffeine is quite safe when used in low doses. The ingestion of a cup of coffee contains, on average, 40–150 mg of caffeine. In large doses, it can be profoundly toxic, resulting in arrhythmia, tachycardia, vomiting, convulsions, coma, and death. The lethal dose occurs with ingestion above 5 g [87].

Indomethacin It consists of a non-steroidal anti-inflammatory, derived from indoleacetic acid. It was first synthesized in 1963, by Shen and collaborators, at the Merck Sharp laboratory [72]. It differs slightly from other anti-inflammatory drugs in its indications and toxic effects. Its mechanism of action is to non-selectively inhibit the enzyme cyclooxygenase, which is necessary for the formation of prostaglandins and thromboxanes. It can also inhibit phospholipases A and C.

Indomethacin is commonly prescribed for the treatment of many primary headaches, such as primary stabbing headache, primary cough headache, primary physical exertion headache, primary headache associated with sexual activity, continuous hemicrania, and paroxysmal hemicrania. These last two are fully responsive to indomethacin [24].

Due to this good response of indomethacin in many primary headaches, it is argued that it should also be used as an alternative in the treatment of hypnic headache [43] and that this headache is classified as an indomethacin-responsive headache [70].

In the cases described, indomethacin was tested in 70 patients, at a dose of 25–200 mg at bedtime, and the response rate found was equal to 50.7%. It is important for the physician to be cautious when prescribing indomethacin to elderly patients because of the adverse effects of this drug [60, 82].

It is assumed that its mechanism of action is by decreasing the pressure of the cerebrospinal fluid (CSF) [88]. The authors observed that indomethacin is particularly beneficial in patients with hypnic headache when the headache attacks are unilateral or patients with associated autonomic features [21, 82].

Other Drugs Despite the good therapeutic response to lithium carbonate, many patients experienced intolerable adverse reactions to this drug or drug interactions that required discontinuation of treatment [12, 15, 36, 39, 42, 46, 52, 54, 55]. Other patients refused to use it because they feared possible side effects [19, 23, 38, 42].

Alternatively, other drugs are used that commonly treat other primary headaches, especially migraine. Among them are melatonin, beta-adrenergic blockers, antidepressants, neuromodulators and / or antiepileptics, calcium channel blockers, serotonergic antagonists, prednisone, etc.

Melatonin or N-acetyl-5-methoxytryptamine is a hormone secreted by the pineal gland, but it is chemically an indolamine synthesized from tryptophan. Its secretion occurs cyclically, as daytime production is minimal, but in the afternoon it increases, peaking between two and six in the morning [89].

The pineal gland participates in the temporal organization of biological rhythms, acting as a mediator between the environmental light / dark cycle and the physiological regulatory processes, including endocrine regulation of reproduction, regulation of activity / rest and sleep / wake cycles, and regulation of the immune system, among others [89].

Some headaches have a clear seasonal and circadian pattern, such as hypnic headache, cyclic migraine, and cluster headache. On the other hand, there is great evidence that headaches are related to pineal gland function and melatonin secretion, as levels of this hormone have been found to be reduced in migraine and cluster headache [90].

The treatment of headaches with melatonin or its agonists is promising and there is great potential for its use in this indication [90]. Possibly, it is a therapeutic option, along with lithium, caffeine, and indomethacin.

There are several cases of hypnic headache treated with melatonin, at a dose of 2 mg–15 mg daily, with a response rate equal to 50% [3, 10, 14, 15, 27, 34, 35, 38, 66]. There is also an isolated case with the use of ramelteon, at a dose of 8 mg daily, a selective agonist of melatonin receptors MT_1 and MT_2, commonly used in the treatment of insomnia. This patient became headache-free for more than 6 months [25].

Beta-adrenergic blockers, such as propranolol and atenolol, which are commonly effective in several primary headaches, have been tried through two possible mechanisms: antagonism to 5-HT_2 receptors or modulating adrenoreceptors. However, they showed no benefit in hypnic headache, presenting a low response rate equal to 27.8% [3, 8, 12, 30, 36–38, 41, 49, 70–72].

In the therapeutic class of antidepressants, both tricyclic and selective serotonin reuptake inhibitors (SSRIs) were used. No therapeutic response was obtained with the use of SSRIs, according to reports of failure with fluoxetine [37, 40], sertraline [27], venlafaxine [37], citalopram [19], trazodone [27], and duloxetina [3]. Of the tricyclic antidepressants, amitriptyline, imipramine, and doxepine have been used in many patients. Amitriptyline, prescribed in 50 patients, was the only drug that showed some efficacy, but with a slight reduction in pain intensity, giving a response rate equal to 22% [3, 8, 21, 35, 57, 73, 74].

Tricyclics act by inhibiting pre-synaptic reuptake of norepinephrine and serotonin. In primary headaches, especially migraine and tension-type headache, there is a good therapeutic response to amitriptyline. However, in hypnic headache, since its first description, its ineffectiveness has been found [70].

Several antiepileptics and/or neuromodulators have been used to treat hypnic headache, including topiramate, gabapentin, lamotrigine, pregabalin, carbamazepine, valproic acid, and sodium divalproate.

Topiramate, a monosaccharide derived from D-fructose, reverses neuronal hyperexcitability, both by increasing GABA-ergic activity and by blocking calcium, chlorine and AMPA glutamate receptors [91]. It has a proven anti-migraine action [89]. In hypnic headache, it was used to treat 31 patients, at a dose of 25 mg–100 mg/day and had a response rate of 41.9% [3, 14, 15, 35, 53, 57, 63, 67].

Gabapentin [3, 28, 34, 37, 38, 62], lamotrigine [5, 32], and pregabalin [34] are possibly effective drugs, but were prescribed in a very small sample, respectively, in nine, three, and one patients. The last two drugs were effective in all patients. Other antiepileptics have shown no therapeutic response. There was failure with carbamazepine [36, 49], valproic acid [36], and sodium valproate [29, 30, 49].

Calcium channel blockers act by selectively blocking the entrance of Ca^{++} into the cell. Of this group, flunarizine and verapamil are used, respectively, in the prophylaxis of migraine and cluster headache. The mechanism of action in headache is unclear. It appears to act to block platelet serotonin release and promote interference with neurovascular inflammation.

Flunarizine and verapamil have been used in prophylaxis of hypnic headache, but with very low efficacy, respectively, of 40.4% and 27.3%. This effect is believed to be related to the activation of D_2 dopaminergic receptors [66].

There are descriptions of several patients who showed a good response to flunarizine [8, 44, 63, 64, 66, 68, 69], at a dose of 2.5 mg–10 mg daily; and to verapamil, at a dose of 240 mg–320 mg daily [21]. It is important to highlight the time they remained asymptomatic [49]. However, there is no reference regarding the time of use of these medications, especially flunarizine. Since most patients are elderly and long-term use can cause secondary parkinsonism.

Serotonergic antagonists are effective in treating migraine, but pizotifene has been shown to be ineffective in hypnic headache [10, 36–38, 49]. However, oxetorone, also a serotonin antagonist and alpha blocker used with an anti-migraine drug, was effective in eight patients [16].

A combination of treatments has been tested, such as, for example, acetazolamide [28, 92], prednisone [9, 12, 18, 27, 28, 38], hypnotics [26], continuous positive airway pressure (CPAP) [27], with partial responses or complete pain remission, but in isolated case reports.

Other types of treatments were used in four patients and can be considered as new therapeutic options. They underwent treatment with botulinum toxin and greater occipital nerve block. Physicians must be cautious about the possible complications of such invasive therapies [82].

The first two patients used botulinum toxin. There was a marked improvement in headache frequency and intensity in only one of them. This patient became asymptomatic in a 12-month follow-up after the second application [19, 67]. A third patient who had refractory hypnic headache underwent nerve stimulation of the occipital nerve and had a good response and consistent effect over 36 months of follow-up [93]. The fourth patient, who had not responded to drug treatment, experienced pain relief with the greater occipital nerve block [14].

Effectiveness of Prophylaxis

In the preventive treatment of hypnic headache, there is a huge therapeutic arsenal and some drugs are classified as being of first choice because they present the best response in pain control. According to the therapeutic response and the size of the sample that benefited from the treatment, the possibility or probability of effectiveness can be expressed (Table 9.3).

Probably effective are the drugs of first choice, those that have been well tested and that the expected effect will happen, such as lithium carbonate, caffeine, indomethacin, and melatonin. While the possibly effective ones may manifest their effect, depending on the sample size, such as, for example, topiramate, lamotrigine, gabapentin, and flunarizine, which have shown some efficacy, but are used in a small number of patients.

On the other hand, some drugs were subsequently tested, without promoting any pain relief, proving to be probably ineffective, whose expected effect will not happen. In this group, there are beta-blockers, tricyclics, SSRIs, verapamil, pizotifene, valproic acid, and sodium valproate.

There are also other treatments tested on a single patient which have shown promise, requiring further studies, such as botulinum toxin, nerve stimulation, and nerve block. In that case, they will be considered as future treatment options.

Follow-Up

The follow-up of the hypnic headache patient for a certain period of time is important to reduce errors with medications, which implies the effectiveness of the treatment and the improvement of the quality of life.

A sample of 97 patients with hypnic headache described in several case series was analyzed, which included three or more patients and who had a follow-up longer than 5 months [94]. The effectiveness was classified according to the statements of the respective authors. In this sample, the follow-up periods of each patient were determined. Then, it was possible to verify whether the headache persisted or disappeared, with or without treatment. In addition, if there was pain recurrence (Table 9.4).

Table 9.4 Follow-up of hypnic headache patients

Authors	n	Remission without treatment	Remission with treatment		Without remission	Follow-up period (years)
			No recurrence	With recurrence		
Raskin 1988 [70]	6	0	3	0	3	4.7 ± 2.9
Morales-Asín et al. 1998 [44]	3	0	2	1	0	1.1 ± 0.8
Dodick et al. 1998 [12]	17	1	4	0	12	3.6 ± 1.5
Pinto et al. 2002 [8]	8	0	1	0	7	NA
Ghiotto et al. 2002 [38]	7	0	0	1	6	NA
Evers et al. 2003 [21]	4	0	0	0	4	NA
Lisotto et al. 2004 [7]	4	0	1	3	0	2.5 ± 1.1
Fukuhara et al. 2006 [33]	3	0	3	0	0	NA
Liang et al., 2008 [54]	17	0	9	5	3	4.2 ± 2.3
Porta-Etessam et al. 2013 [64]	6	0	6	0	0	NA
Silva-Néto et al. 2014 [72]	22	0	11	5	6	≥ 0.5
TOTAL (n; %)	97 (100%)	1 (1%)	40 (41.2)	15 (15.5)	41 (42.3)	

NA: Not available

Source: Silva-Néto RP, Sousa-Santos PEM, Peres MFP. Hypnic headache: A review of 348 cases published from 1988 to 2018. J Neurol Sci 2019;401:103-9

Prognosis and Complications

There was not a large number of patients treated so far, but from the analysis of 97 cases that were followed, it is concluded that 1% of patients have remission without treatment and 56.7% will be free of pain with effective treatment. However, more than 40% will experience no remission of pain and will continue to experience headache chronically [94]. One study revealed that 53% of patients enter an episodic course after treatment [95]. Although most patients diagnosed with hypnic headache have a good therapeutic response, some authors believe that hypnic headache is a chronic disorder and can occur for many years without headache remission [1].

There are no long-term neurological complications in patients with hypnic headache, as most experience pain relief after treatment. Some outcomes of hypnic headache are well known. If diagnosed correctly, patients will have a good outcome, but relapses are not uncommon. Debilitating effects of occasional severe headache attacks are limited and can be easily aborted [2].

References

1. Liang JF, Wang SJ. Hypnic headache: a review of clinical features, therapeutic options and outcomes. Cephalalgia. 2014;34(10):795–805.
2. Tariq N, Estemalik E, Vij B, Kriegler JS, Tepper SJ, Stillman MJ. Long-term outcomes and clinical characteristics of hypnic headache syndrome: 40 patients series from a tertiary referral center. Headache. 2016;56(4):717–24.
3. Bender SD. An unusual case of hypnic headache ameliorated utilizing a mandibular advancement oral appliance. Sleep Breath. 2012;16(3):599–602.
4. Ouahmane Y, Mounach J, Satte A, Zerhouni A, Ouhabi H. Hypnic headache: response to lamotrigine in two cases. Cephalalgia. 2012;32(8):645–8.
5. Baykan B, Ertas M. Hypnic headache associated with medication overuse: case report. Agri. 2008;20(3):40–3.
6. Lisoto C, Mainardi F, Maggioni F, Zanchin G. Episodic hypnic headache? Cephalalgia. 2004;24(8):681–5.
7. Pinto CAR, Fragoso YD, Souza Carvalho D, Gabbai AA. Hypnic headache syndrome: clinical aspects of eight patients in Brazil. Cephalalgia. 2002;22(10):824–7.
8. Relja G, Zorzon M, Locatelli L, Carraro N, Antonello RM, Cazzato G. Hypnic headache: rapid and long-lasting response to prednisone in two new cases. Cephalalgia. 2002;22(2):157–9.
9. Capo G, Esposito A. Hypnic headache. A new Italian case with a good response to pizotifene and melatonin (abstract). Proceedings of 10th congress of the international headache society, 2001 Jun 29 to Jul 3; New York, EUA. Cephalalgia. 2001;21(4):505–6.
10. Martins IP, Gouveia RG. Hypnic headache and travel across time zones: a case report. Cephalalgia. 2001;21(9):928–31.
11. Dodick DW, Mosek AC, Campbell JK. The hypnic ('alarm clock') headache syndrome. Cephalalgia. 1998;18(3):152–6.
12. Pinto CAR, Fragoso YD, Souza Carvalho D, Gabbai AA. Síndrome da cefaleia hípnica: aspectos clínicos de 16 pacientes. Rev Neurociênc. 2003;11(1):46–51.
13. Rehmann R, Tegenthoff M, Zimmer C, Stude P. Case report of an alleviation of pain symptoms in hypnic headache via greater occipital nerve block. Cephalalgia. 2017;37(10):998–1000.
14. Holle D, Wessendorf TE, Zaremba S, Naegel S, Diener HC, Katsarava Z, et al. Serial polysomnography in hypnic headache. Cephalalgia. 2011;31(3):286–90.
15. Donnet A, Lantéri-Minet M. A consecutive series of 22 cases of hypnic headache in France. Cephalalgia. 2009;29(9):928–34.
16. Centonze V, D'Amico D, Usai S, Causarano V, Bassi A, Bussone G. First Italian case of hypnic headache, with literature review and discussion of nosology. Cephalalgia. 2001;21(1):71–4.
17. Zanchin G, Lisotto C, Maggioni F. The hypnic headache syndrome: the first description of an Italian case. J Headache Pain. 2000;1(1):60.
18. Marziniak M, Voss J, Evers S. Hypnic headache successfully treated with botulinum toxin type a. Cephalalgia. 2007;27(9):1082–4.
19. Evans RW, Dodick DW, Schwedt TJ. The headaches that awaken us. Headache. 2006;46(4):678–81.
20. Evers S, Rahmann A, Schwaag S, Lüdermann P, Husstedt IW. Hypnic headache – the first German cases including polysomnography. Cephalalgia. 2003;23(1):20–3.

21. Peters N, Lorenzl S, Fischereder J, Bötzel K, Straube A. Hypnic headache: a case presentation including polysomnography. Cephalalgia. 2006;26(1):84–6.
22. Peng H, Wang L, He B, Giudice M, Zhang L, Zhao ZX. Hypnic headache responsive to sodium ferulate in 2 new cases. Clin J Pain. 2013;29(1):89–91.
23. Goadsby PJ, Lipton RB. A review of paroxysmal hemicranias, SUNCT syndrome and other short-lasting headaches with autonomic feature, including new cases. Brain. 1997;120(1):193–209.
24. Arai M. A case of unilateral hypnic headache: rapid response to ramelteon, a selective melatonin MT1/MT2 receptor agonist. Headache. 2015;55(7):1010–1.
25. Dodick DW, Jones JM, Capobianco DJ. Hypnic headache: another indomethacin-responsive headache syndrome? Headache. 2000;40(10):830–5.
26. Karlovasitou A, Avdelidi E, Andriopoulou G, Baloyannis S. Transient hypnic headache syndrome in a patient with bipolar disorder after the withdrawal of long-term lithium treatment: a case report. Cephalalgia. 2009;29(4):484–6.
27. Schürks M, Kastrup O, Diener HC. Triptan responsive hypnic headache? Eur J Neurol. 2006;13(6):666–72.
28. Dissanayake KP, Wanniarachchi DP, Ranawaka UK. Case report of hypnic headache: a rare headache disorder with nocturnal symptoms. BMC Res Notes. 2017;10(1):318.
29. Prakash S, Dahbi AS. Relapsing remitting hypnic headache responsive to indomethacin in an adolescent: a case report. J Headache Pain. 2008;9(6):393–5.
30. Aguirre-Rodríguez CJ, Hernández-Martínez N, Aguirre-Rodríguez FJ. Cefalea hípnica, a propósito de un caso. SEMERGEN. 2016;42(2):12–3.
31. Fantini J, Granato A, Zorzon M, Manganotti P. Case report: coexistence of SUNCT and hypnic headache in the same patient. Headache. 2016;56(9):1503–6.
32. Fukuhara Y, Takeshima T, Ishizaki K, Burioka N, Nakashima K. Three Japanese cases of hypnic headache. Rinsho Shinkeigaku. 2006;46(2):148–53.
33. Ulrich K, Gunreben B, Lang E, Sitti R, Griessinger N. Pregabalin in the therapy of hypnic headache. Cephalalgia. 2006;26(8):1031–2.
34. Jiménez-Caballero PE, Gámez-Leyva G, Gómez M, Casado-Naranjo I. Descripción de una serie de casos de cefalea hípnica. Diferenciación entre sexos. Rev Neurol. 2012;54(6):332–6.
35. Guido M, Specchio LM. Successful treatment of hypnic headache with topiramate: a case report. Headache. 2006;46(7):1205–6.
36. Arjona JA, Jimenez-Jimenez FJ, Vela-Bueno A, Tallon-Barranco A. Hypnic headache associated with stage 3 slow wave sleep. Headache. 2000;40(9):753–4.
37. Ghiotto N, Sances G, Di Lorenzo G, Trucco M, Loi M, Sandrini G, et al. Report of eight new cases of hypnic headache and mini-review of the literature. Funct Neurol. 2002;17(4):211–9.
38. Garza I, Swanson J. Successful preventive therapy in hypnic headache using hypnotics: a case report. Cephalalgia. 2007;27(9):1080–1.
39. Raskin NH. The hypnic headache syndrome. Headache. 1988;28(8):534–6.
40. Queiroz LP, Coral LC. The hypnic headache syndrome – a case report (Abstract). Proceedings of 8th Congress of the International Headache Society, 1997 Jun 10–14; Amsterdam, Germany. Cephalalgia. 1997;17(3):303.
41. Skobieranda FG, Lee TG, Solomon GD. The hypnic headache syndrome: six additional patients (abstract). Proceedings of 8th congress of the international headache society, 1997 Jun 10-14; Amsterdam, Germany. Cephalalgia. 1997;17(3):304–5.
42. Ivañez V, Soler R, Barreiro P. Hypnic headache syndrome: a case with good response to indomethacin. Cephalalgia. 1998;18(4):225–6.
43. Morales-Asín F, Mauri JA, Iñiguez C, Espada F, Mostacero E. The hypnic headache syndrome: report of three new cases. Cephalalgia. 1998;18(3):157–8.
44. Perez-Martinez DA, Berbel-Garcia A, Puente-Muñoz AI, Saiz-Diaz RA, de Toledo-Heras M, Porta-Etessam J, et al. Hypnic headache: a new case. Rev Neurol. 1999;28(9):883–4.
45. Trucco M, Maggioni F, Badino R, Zanchin G. Hypnic headache syndrome: report of a new Italian case. Cephalalgia. 2000;20(4):312.

46. Vieira-Dias M, Esperança P. Hypnic headache: report of two cases. Headache. 2001;41(7):726–7.
47. Brooks PT, Hadjikoutis S, Pickersgill TP. Lithium responsive hypnic headache in a patient with multiple sclerosis (Abstract). Proceedings of Association of British Neurologists Spring Meeting, 2003 Apr 2–4; Cardiff, UK. J Neurol Neurosurg Psychiatry. 2003;74(10):1459.
48. Pinessi L, Rainero I, Cicolin A, Zibetti M, Gentile S, Mutani R. Hypnic headache syndrome: association of the attacks with REM sleep. Cephalalgia. 2003;23(2):150–4.
49. Kocasoy-Orhan E, Kayrak-Ertas N, Orhan KS, Ertas M. Hypnic headache syndrome: excessive periodic limb movements in polysomnography. Agri. 2004;16(4):28–30.
50. Patsouros N, Laloux P, Ossemann M. Hypnic headache: a case report with polysomnography. Acta Neurol Belg. 2004;104(1):37–40.
51. Kerr E, Hewitt R, Gleadhill I. Benign headache in the elderly – a case report of hypnic headache. Ulster Med J. 2006;75(2):158–9.
52. Autunno M, Messina C, Blandino A, Rodolico C. Hypnic headache responsive to low-dose topiramate: a case report. Headache. 2008;48(2):292–4.
53. Liang JF, Fuh JL, Yu HY, Hsu CY, Wang SJ. Clinical features, polysomnography and outcome in patients with hypnic headache. Cephalalgia. 2008;28(3):209–15.
54. Caminero AB, Martín J, Del Río MS. Secondary hypnic headache or symptomatic nocturnal hipertensión? Two case reports. Cephalalgia. 2010;30(9):1137–9.
55. Silva-Néto RP, Almeida KJ. Hypnic headache: a descriptive study of 25 new cases in Brazil. J Neurol Sci. 2014;338(1–2):166–8.
56. Pérez Hernández A, Gómez OE. Influenza a virus: a possible trigger factor for hypnic headache? Neurologia. 2017;32(1):67–8.
57. Zhang Y, Wang C, Chen Y, Wang R, Lian Y. Hypnic headache with dopaminergic neuron dysfunction: new insight from a rare case. Pain Med. 2019;20(8):1639–42.
58. Manni R, Sances G, Terzaghi M, Ghiotto N, Nappi G. Hypnic headache: PSG evidence of both REM-and NREM-related attacks. Neurology. 2004;62(8):1411–3.
59. Buzzi MG, Cologno D, Formisano R, Caltagirone C. Hypnic headache responsive to indomethacin: second Italian case. Funct Neurol. 2005;20(2):85–7.
60. Seidel S, Zeitlhofer J, Wöber C. First Austrian case of hypnic headache: serial polysomnography and blood pressure monitoring in treatment with indomethacin. Cephalalgia. 2008;28(10):1086–90.
61. Porta-Etessam JP, García-Morales I, Di Capua D, García-Cobos R. A patient with primary sexual headache associated with hypnic headaches. J Headache Pain. 2009;10(2):135.
62. Dolezil D, Mavrokordatos C. Hypnic headache- a rare primary headache disorder with very good response to indomethacin. Neuro Endocrinol Lett. 2012;33(6):597–9.
63. Mulero P, Guerrero-Peral AL, Cortijo E, Jabary NS, Herrero-Velázquez S, Miranda S, et al. Cefalea hípnica: características de una serie de 13 nuevos casos y propuesta de modificación de los criterios diagnósticos. Rev Neurol. 2012;54(3):129–36.
64. Porta-Etessam J, Muñiz S, Cuadrado ML, González-García N, Orviz A, Abarrategui B, et al. Successful treatment of hypnic headache syndrome with flunarizine. J Neurol Neurosci. 2013;(4)1:2.
65. Escudero Martínez I, González-Oria C, Bernal Sánchez-Arjona M, Jiménez Hernández MD. Description of series of 10 patients with hypnic headache: discussion of the diagnostic criteria. Neurologia. 2015;30(4):195–200.
66. Domitrz I. Hypnic headache as a primary short-lasting night headache: a report of two cases. Neurol Neurochir Pol. 2005;39(1):77–9.
67. Kesserwani H. Hypnic headache responds to topiramate: a case report and a review of mechanisms of action of therapeutic agents. Cureus. 2021;13(3):13790.
68. Klimek A, Sklodowski P, Night headache. Report of 2 cases. Neurol Neurochir Pol. 1999;33(5):49–54.
69. Porta-Etessam J, Pérez-Martínez DA, Martínez-Salio A, Berbel-García A, Gordo R. Successful treatment of hypnic headache syndrome with flunarizine (Abstract). Proceedings of 8th Headache Congress of the European Headache Federation, 2006 Apr 26–29; Valencia, Spain. J Headache Pain. 2006;7(1):56.

70. Gould JD, Silberstein SD. Unilateral hypnic headache: a case study. Neurology. 1997;49(6):1749–51.
71. Evers S, Goadsby PJ. Hypnic headache. Pract Neurol. 2005;5(3):144–9.
72. Silva-Néto RP, Bernardino SN. Ambulatory blood pressure monitoring in patient with hypnic headache: a case study. Headache. 2013;53(7):1157–8.
73. Capuano A, Vollono C, Rubino M, Mei D, Cali C, De Angelis A, et al. Hypnic headache: actigraphic and polysomnographic study of a case. Cephalalgia. 2005;25(6):466–9.
74. Dolso P, Merlino G, Fratticci L, Canesin R, Valiante G, Coccolo D, et al. Non-REM hypnic headache: a circadian disorder? A clinical and polysomnography. Cephalalgia. 2006;27(1):83–6.
75. Silva-Néto RP, Roesler CP, Raffaelli E Jr. Nocturnal headache, nightmares and lithium. Migrâneas Cefaleias. 2008;11(1):14–6.
76. Silva-Néto R. Cefaleias noturnas. In: Silva-Néto R, editor. Cefaleia – aspectos históricos e tópicos relevantes. Teresina: Halley; 2013. p. 139–44.
77. Chazot G, Claustrat B, Brun J, Zaidan R. Effects of the patterns of melatonin and cortisol in cluster headache of a single administration of lithium at 7:00 p.m. daily over one week: a preliminary report. Pharmacopsychiatry. 1987;20:222–3.
78. Lewis AJ, Kerenyi NA, Feuer G. Neuropharmacology of pineal secretion. Drug Metabol Drug Interact. 1990;8(3–4):247–312.
79. Pablos MI, Santaolaya MJ, Agapito MT, Recio JM. Influence of lithium salts on chick pineal gland melatonin secretion. Neurosci Lett. 1994;174(1):55–7.
80. Treiser SL, Cascio CS, O'Donohue TL, Thoa NB, Jacobowitz DM, Kellar KJ. Lithium increases serotonin release and decreases serotonin receptors in the hippocampus. Science. 1981;213(4515):1529–31.
81. Newman LC, Lipton RB, Solomon S. The hypnic headache syndrome: a benign headache disorder of the elderly. Neurology. 1990;40(12):1904–5.
82. Al Khalili Y, Chopra P. Hypnic headache. In: StatPearls [internet]. Treasure Island. Florida: StatPearls Publishing; 2022.
83. Morales F. Síndrome de cefalea hípnica. Revisión Rev Soc Esp Dolor. 1999;6(5):363–7.
84. Waldvogel SR. Caffeine - a drug with a surprise. Angew Chem Int Ed Engl. 2003;42(6):604–5.
85. Mathew RJ, Wilson WH. Caffeine induced changes in cerebral circulation. Stroke. 1985;16(5):814–7.
86. Silva-Néto RP, Soares AA. O papel da cafeína nas cefaléias: fator agravante ou atenuante? Migrâneas cefaleias. 2006;9(3):72–7.
87. Kerrigan S, Lindsey T. Fatal caffeine overdose: two case reports. Forensic Sci Int. 2005;153(1):67–9.
88. Diener HC, Obermann M, Holle D. Hypnic headache: clinical course and treatment. Curr Treat Options Neurol. 2012;14(1):15–26.
89. Borjigin J, Zhang LS, Calinescu AA. Circadian regulation of pineal gland rhythmicity. Mol Cell Endocrinol. 2012;349(1):13–9.
90. Peres MF, Masruha MR, Zukerman E, Moreira-Filho CA, Cavalheiro EA. Potential therapeutic use of melatonin in migraine and other headache disorders. Expert Opin Investig Drugs. 2006;15(4):367–75.
91. Ferrari A, Tiraferri I, Neri L, Sternieri E. Clinical pharmacology of topiramate in migraine prevention. Expert Opin Drug Metab Toxicol. 2011;7(9):1169–81.
92. Sibon I, Ghorayeb I, Henry P. Successful treatment of hypnic headache syndrome with acetazolamide. Neurology. 2003;61(8):1157–8.
93. Son BC, Yang SH, Hong JT, Lee SW. Occipital nerve stimulation for medically refractory hypnic headache. Neuromodulation. 2012;15(4):381–6.
94. Silva-Néto RP, Sousa-Santos PEM, Peres MFP. Hypnic headache: a review of 348 cases published from 1988 to 2018. J Neurol Sci. 2019;15(401):103–9.
95. Evers S, Goadsby PJ. Hypnic headache: clinical features, pathophysiology, and treatment. Neurology. 2003;60(6):905–9.

Chapter 10
A New Classification for Hypnic Headache

They say pain makes us wise

Alfred Tennyson (1809-1892)

Introduction

In 2004, hypnic headache was included for the first time in the classification of headaches. One of the diagnostic criteria was that the headache could occur >15 times a month [1]. However, current diagnostic criteria for hypnic headache are: developing only during sleep, and causing awakening of patient; occurring on ≥10 days/ month, for >3 months; lasting from 15 mins up to 4 h after waking; and no cranial autonomic symptoms or restlessness [2].

Based on the authors' experience, it has been observed that most patients with hypnic headache have more than 15 headache days per month. Hypnic headache could be classified into episodic and chronic forms, following the same criteria as other primary headaches, such as migraine, tension-type headache, and cluster headache.

Episodic and Chronic Forms

Based on the last hypnic headache review that described 343 adult patients from 1988 to 2018 [3] and two more that were published in the period from 2019 to 2022 [4, 5], the monthly frequency of headache attacks of the 345 adult patients was analyzed.

Of the 345 patients, only 305 provided information on the frequency of headache attacks. They were divided into two groups: in-group 1, frequency < 15 days per

R. Silva-Néto, D. Holle-Lee, *Hypnic Headache*,
https://doi.org/10.1007/978-3-031-32263-1_10

month; and in-group 2, frequency ≥ 15 days per month, and named, respectively, episodic hypnic headache (EHH) and chronic hypnic headache (CHH).

In only 57.7% (176/305) of the selected patients, there was information about sex, age at onset of pain, latency until diagnosis, and clinical characterization of headache. There were no details of this information in five large series of patients who have been diagnosed with EHH or CHH [6–10]. The selected sample comprised 176 patients who were divided into 43 with HHE and 133 with CHH.

There were 176 hypnic headache patients with a mean age at pain onset of 59.8 ± 12.8 in age and ranging from 15 to 85 years. Forty-three patients (24.4%) had a frequency of headache attacks <15 days per month and 133 (75.6%), ≥15 days per month. EHH affected patients aged 57.3 ± 12.2 years, while in CHH, the age was 60.8 ± 12.9 years (not significant), as shown in Table 10.1.

The distribution of the clinical characteristics of 176 patients with hypnic headache is summarized in Table 10.2.

In assessing the therapeutic response to preventive treatment, only drugs reported in at least three patients were considered. Drug efficacies were classified according to authors' statements. Lithium, caffeine, indomethacin, and melatonin were considered effective options for preventive treatment (Table 10.3).

From two comparison groups, headache features of 176 patients described with hypnic headache in the last 34 years were analyzed. The objective was to identify whether these features justify dividing hypnic headache into chronic versus episodic forms, by headache frequency dichotomized on 15 days per month.

In the first diagnostic criteria for hypnic headache suggested by Goadsby and Lipton in 1997, the headache could occur at least 15 days per month for at least 1 month [11]. In 2003, Evers and Goadsby made these criteria more specific than the previous ones. They have been modified, but the number of attacks per month has remained unchanged [12] and they were included in ICHD-2 [1]. In both ICHD-3beta and ICHD-3, criterion C changed to accommodate headaches occurring

Table 10.1 Distribution of sex, age of onset of pain, and latency until diagnosis according to frequency of headache attacks in 43 patients with EHH and 133 with CHH

Variables	Diagnosis		*p* Value
	EHH	CHH	
Sex			0.781[a]
Female (*n*; %)	32 (74.4)	94 (70.7)	
Male (*n*; %)	11 (25.6)	39 (29.3)	
Age of onset of pain (years)			0.128[b]
Average (SD)	57.3 (12.2)	60.8 (12.9)	
Variation	28–81	15–85	
Latency until diagnosis (years)			0.740[b]
Average (SD)	4.6 (7.3)	5.1 (6.8)	
Variation	0.3–39.6	0.3–42	

[a]*p*-value based on Chi-square test for mean difference of unpaired samples
[b]Student's t-test p-value for mean difference of unpaired samples
Note: EHH—episodic hypnic headache; CHH—chronic hypnic headache; SD—standard deviation
Source: Silva-Néto. Cefaleia hípnica: Dores que vem pelo sono. Nova Aliança: Teresina, 2019

Table 10.2 Clinical characteristics of 43 patients with episodic hypnic headache and 133 with chronic hypnic headache

	Diagnosis				
	EHH		CHH		
Characteristics	*n*	%	*n*	%	*p* Value
Timing of attacks					0.041
0:00–2:00 a.m.	13	30.2	51	38.4	
2:00–4:00 a.m.	16	37.2	60	45.1	
4:00–6:00 a.m.	14	32.6	22	16.5	
Duration of attacks (minutes)					0.035
< 30	8	18.6	9	6.8	
30–120	25	58.1	96	72.2	
> 120	10	23.3	28	21.0	
Quality of pain					0.014
Dull/pressure	24	55.8	97	72.9	
Stabbing / burning	10	23.3	28	21.1	
Throbbing / pulsatile	9	20.9	8	6.0	
Intensity of pain					0.707
Mild (VRS 1–4)	1	2.3	10	7.5	
Moderate (VRS 5–7)	24	55.8	64	48.1	
Severe (VRS 8–9)	16	37.2	56	42.1	
Very severe (VRS 10)	2	4.7	3	2.3	
Localization of pain					0.009
Bilateral	16	37.2	82	61.6	
Unilateral	17	39.5	34	25.6	
Holocranial / diffuse	10	23.3	17	12.8	
Trigeminal-autonomic features					0.990
Absent	41	95.3	128	96.2	
Present	2	4.7	5	3.8	

Note: EHH—episodic hypnic headache; CHH—chronic hypnic headache; VRS—verbal rating scale
Source: Silva-Néto. Cefaleia hípnica: Dores que vem pelo sono. Nova Aliança: Teresina, 2019

on ≥10 days per month, for more than 3 months [2, 13], because data showed 95% of patients felt in this category [3].

After dividing the patients into two groups (<15 days of pain per month and ≥ 15 days of pain per month), the episodic form was observed in 24.4% and chronic in 75.6%. CHH was the predominant form, in which headache attacks tend to occur in the first hours of sleep, last longer, with a dull or pressure character, and are located bilaterally. None of these differences survived correction for multiple comparisons. This may be because the 15-day dichotomy is not biologically useful or because, in essence, hypnic headache exists on a frequency spectrum.

ICHD-3 establishes a minimum limit of 10 headache days per month. It could be argued that there should be a minimum number of headache attacks. If there is no minimum period, this would not qualify as a disorder. Arbitrarily one could set five

Table 10.3 Drugs used in the prophylactic treatment of patients with episodic hypnic headache or with chronic hypnic headache

	Efficacy										
	Episodic hypnic headache					Chronic hypnic headache					
Treatment	n	None	Partial (A)	Good (B)	Response rate (A + B/n, %)	n	None	Partial (A)	Good (B)	Response rate (A + B/n, %)	*p* Value
Lithium	14	4	–	10	71.4	48	8	2	38	83.3	0.442
Caffeine	–	–	–	–	–	20	5	3	12	75.0	NA
Indomethacin	9	2	1	6	77.8	33	11	2	19	63.6	0.693
Melatonin	1	–	–	1	100.0	7	2	–	5	71.4	NA
Topiramate	4	–	3	1	100.0	4	1	–	2	50.0	NA
Flunarizine	2	–	–	2	100.0	23	8	7	8	65.2	NA
Beta-blockers	–	–	–	–	–	14	13	–	1	7.1	NA
Tricyclic antidepressants	2	–	–	2	100.0	23	20	1	2	13.0	NA
Gabapentin	–	–	–	–	–	6	2	–	4	66,7	NA
Prednisone	–	–	–	–	–	4	3	1	–	25.0	NA
Verapamil	–	–	–	–	–	9	6	–	3	33.3	NA
Pizotifen	–	–	–	–	–	6	4	–	2	33.3	NA
SSRIs	–	–	–	–	–	5	5	–	–	0.0	NA
Lamotrigine	–	–	–	–	–	3	–	–	3	100.0	NA

Note: NA—not applicable; SSRIs—selective serotonin reuptake inhibitors
Source: Silva-Néto. Cefaleia hípnica: Dores que vem pelo sono. Nova Aliança: Teresina, 2019

Table 10.4 Proposal for a new classification for hypnic headache

Episodic hypnic headache	Chronic hypnic headache
A. At least five recurrent headache attacks fulfilling criteria B–E B. Developing only during sleep, and causing wakening C. Occurring on <15 days/month for >3 months D. Lasting from 15 mins up to 4 h after waking E. no cranial autonomic symptoms or restlessness F. Not better accounted for by another ICHD-3 diagnosis	A. At least five recurrent headache attacks fulfilling criteria B–E B. Developing only during sleep, and causing wakening C. Occurring on ≥15 days/month for >3 months D. Lasting from 15 mins up to 4 h after waking E. no cranial autonomic symptoms or restlessness F. Not better accounted for by another ICHD-3 diagnosis

Source: Silva-Néto. Cefaleia hípnica: Dores que vem pelo sono. Nova Aliança: Teresina, 2019

attacks, as is used in migraine as an "A" level criterion. One possible classification for the disorder is presented in Table 10.4. It could be argued that the cut-point for EHH should reflect disability and utility of preventive therapy. This is widely considered to sit at about 4 days a month for migraine.

Allowing an episodic form for hypnic headache may disclose new cases not previously reported because it would not fit current diagnostic criteria. Interestingly, the prevalence study performed in Iceland, found two probable hypnic headache cases out of 921 individuals, the criteria not fulfilled was exactly "number of headaches higher than 10 per month." [14] Episodic primary headaches are more common than chronic forms, but it seems to be different for hypnic headache.

Regarding treatment options, no changes were observed in responses reported by authors for the current options available, which are lithium, caffeine, indomethacin, and melatonin in episodic or chronic forms. However, a lack of randomized clinical trials limits the validity of this information [1, 3].

Limitations for a Classification

An important and fundamental limitation is the reliance, without scrutiny of original material, on published case series. Patients with nocturnal onset migraine who have a typical migraine phenotype and less bothersome attacks at other times may be labelled as hypnic headache. It could be argued that the small series have limits of experience, and equally that the large series over-diagnose the condition. This is an almost unresolvable problem with research in rare headache disorders.

Absent a biomarker evolving or an understanding of the basis for the effect of either lithium or caffeine, which seem to be the standards in therapy, progress will be hindered. One such consideration would be the effect of both lithium [15] and caffeine [16], which increase slow wave sleep [17], remarkably for caffeine in the same epoch [16] as the most common occurrence for hypnic headache attacks [18]. This is unclear for indomethacin [19]. Whether 15 is the correct frequency, a dichotomy provides an additional limit to the study. There is even emerging evidence and opinion that fifteen is not the ideal distinction in frequency for migraine [20]. Perhaps the search for the correct point of dichotomy is our Ulysses odyssey.

The authors believe hypnic headache could be classified into episodic or chronic forms. However, further studies are needed to clarify the hypnic headache phenotype and its prevalence in the general population. Whether further studies support that distinction, less frequent forms of hypnic headache can be studied and the prevalence of all forms in the general population can be understood.

References

1. Headache Classification Subcommittee of the International Headache Society. The international classification of headache disorders, 2nd edition. Cephalalgia. 2004;24(1):8–160.
2. Headache Classification Subcommittee of the International Headache Society. The International Classification of Headache Disorders, 3rd edition. Cephalalgia. 2018;38(1):1–211.
3. Silva-Néto RP, Sousa-Santos PEM, Peres MFP. Hypnic headache: a review of 348 cases published from 1988 to 2018. J Neurol Sci. 2019;401:103–9.

4. Zhang Y, Wang C, Chen Y, Wang R, Lian Y. Hypnic headache with dopaminergic neuron dysfunction: new insight from a rare case. Pain Med. 2019;20(8):1639–42.
5. Kesserwani H. Hypnic headache responds to topiramate: a case report and a review of mechanisms of action of therapeutic agents. Cureus. 2021;13(3):13790.
6. Dodick DW, Mosek AC, Campbell JK. The hypnic ('alarm clock') headache syndrome. Cephalalgia. 1998;18(3):152–6.
7. Liang JF, Fuh JL, Yu HY, Hsu CY, Wang SJ. Clinical features, polysomnography and outcome in patients with hypnic headache. Cephalalgia. 2008;28(3):209–15.
8. Donnet A, Lantéri-Minet M. A consecutive series of 22 cases of hypnic headache in France. Cephalalgia. 2009;29(9):928–34.
9. Jiménez-Caballero PE, Gámez-Leyva G, Gómez M, Casado-Naranjo I. Descripción de una serie de casos de cefalea hípnica. Diferenciación entre sexos Rev Neurol. 2012;54(6):332–6.
10. Tariq N, Estemalik E, Vij B, Kriegler JS, Tepper SJ, Stillman MJ. Long-term outcomes and clinical characteristics of hypnic headache syndrome: 40 patients series from a tertiary referral center. Headache. 2016;56(4):717–24.
11. Goadsby PJ, Lipton RB. A review of paroxysmal hemicranias, SUNCT syndrome and other short-lasting headaches with autonomic feature, including new cases. Brain. 1997;120(1):193–209.
12. Evers S, Goadsby PJ. Hypnic headache: clinical features, pathophysiology, and treatment. Neurology. 2003;60(6):905–9.
13. Headache lassification Subcommittee of the International Headache Society. The international classification of headache disorders, 3rd edition (beta version). Cephalalgia. 2013;33(9):629–808.
14. Eliasson JH, Scher AI, Buse DC, Tietjen G, Lipton RB, Launer LJ, et al. The prevalence of hypnic headache in Iceland. Cephalalgia. 2020;40(8):863–5.
15. Friston KJ, Sharpley AL, Solomon RA, Cowen PJ. Lithium increases slow wave sleep: possible mediation by brain 5-HT2 receptors? Psychopharmacology. 1989;98(1):139–40.
16. Paterson LM, Nutt DJ, Ivarsson M, Hutson PH, Wilson SJ. Effects on sleep stages and microarchitecture of caffeine and its combination with zolpidem or trazodone in healthy volunteers. J Psychopharmacol. 2009;23(5):487–94.
17. Nesbitt AD, Leschziner GD, Peatfield RC. Headache, drugs and sleep. Cephalalgia. 2014;34(10):756–66.
18. Holle D, Naegel S, Obermann M. Hypnic headache. Cephalalgia. 2013;33(16):1349–57.
19. Murphy PJ, Badia P, Myers BL, Boecker MR, Wright KP Jr. Nonsteroidal anti-inflammatory drugs affect normal sleep patterns in humans. Physiol Behav. 1994;55(6):1063–6.
20. Ishii R, Schwedt TJ, Dumkrieger G, Lalvani N, Craven A, Goadsby PJ, et al. Chronic versus episodic migraine: the 15-day threshold does not adequately reflect substantial differences in disability across the full spectrum of headache frequency. Headache. 2021;61(7):992–1003.

Chapter 11
Scientific Publications on Hypnic Headache

It is not in science that happiness is, but in the acquisition of science

Edgar Allan Poe (1809–1849)

Introduction

The first scientific article on hypnic headache was published by Raskin 30 years ago, entitled "*The hypnic Headache syndrome*." [1] Since then, more than a hundred articles have been written on all continents, especially in the last 5 years.

Today, doctors of different specialties know hypnic headache all over the world. In medical texts from different areas of medicine, the expression "hypnic headache" is found. A search in the PubMed medical database, on December 31, 2022, using the descriptor "hypnic headache," showed 37,725 results.

In the medical literature, articles indexed in several databases are available that describe case reports, case series, reviews, and updates on this topic, written in English, Spanish, and Portuguese. In addition, there are also book chapters that summarize this knowledge [1–152].

Published cases of hypnic headache come from 21 countries distributed on almost all continents. Most of the cases are from authors from Spain, the USA, Italy, Brazil, Germany, and France. Table 11.1 shows the distribution of 19 authors with ≥4 publications on hypnic headache according to country of origin.

Next, the current references on hypnic headache that made up this book will be presented.

R. Silva-Néto, D. Holle-Lee, *Hypnic Headache*,
https://doi.org/10.1007/978-3-031-32263-1_11

Table 11.1 Distribution of 19 authors with ≥4 publications on hypnic headache according to country of origin

Author	Country of origin	Number of publications
Dagny Holle	Essen (Germany)	11
Mark Obermann	Essen (Germany)	10
Raimundo Silva-Néto	Teresina (Brazil)	10
Hans-Christoph Diener	Essen (Germany)	8
Steffen Naegel	Essen (Germany)	8
David W. Dodick	Scottsdale (USA)	7
Charly Gaul	Essen (Germany)	6
Lipton RB	New York (USA)	5
Giorgio Zanchin	Padua (Italy)	5
Setfan Evers	Münster (Germany)	4
Yara Dadalti Fragoso	Santos (Brazil)	4
Peter J. Goadsby	London (UK)	4
Zaza Katsarava	Essen (Germany)	4
Sarah Krebs	Essen (Germany)	4
Carlo Lisotto	Pordenone (Italy)	4
Ferdinando Maggioni	Padua (Italy)	4
Pinto CAR	São Paulo (Brazil)	4
Jesús Porta-Etessam	Madrid (Spain)	4
Souza Carvalho D	São Paulo (Brazil)	4

Source: Silva-Néto RP, Sousa-Santos PEM, Peres MFP. Hypnic headache: A review of 348 cases published from 1988 to 2018. J Neurol Sci 2019;401:103–9

References

1. Raskin NH. The hypnic headache syndrome. Headache. 1988;28(8):534–6.
2. Aguirre-Rodríguez CJ, Hernández-Martínez N, Aguirre-Rodríguez FJ. Cefalea hípnica, a propósito de un caso. SEMERGEN. 2016;42(2):12–3.
3. Alberti A. Headache and sleep. Sleep Med Rev. 2006;10(6):431–7.
4. Aldred MP, Raviskanthan S, Mortensen PW, Lee AG. Hypnic headaches in a patient post coiling and clipping of intracranial aneurysm. J Neuroophthalmol. 2021;42(1):415–6.
5. Al Khalili Y, Chopra P. Hypnic headache. In: StatPearls [internet]. Treasure Island. Florida: StatPearls Publishing; 2022.
6. Almeida RF, Leão IMT, Gomes JBL. Cefaleia hípnica. Migrâneas e Cefaleias. 2007;10(1):20–3.
7. Arai M. A case of unilateral hypnic headache: rapid response to ramelteon, a selective melatonin MT1/MT2 receptor agonist. Headache. 2015;55(7):1010–1.
8. Autunno M, Messina C, Blandino A, Rodolico C. Hypnic headache responsive to low-dose topiramate: a case report. Headache. 2008;48(2):292–4.
9. Baykan B, Ertas M. Hypnic headache associated with medication overuse: case report. Agri. 2008;20(3):40–3.
10. Bender SD. An unusual case of hypnic headache ameliorated utilizing a mandibular advancement oral appliance. Sleep Breath. 2012;16(3):599–602.
11. Brooks PT, Hadjikoutis S, Pickersgill TP. Lithium responsive hypnic headache in a patient with multiple sclerosis (Abstract). Proceedings of Association of British Neurologists Spring Meeting, 2003 Apr 2–4; Cardiff, UK. J Neurol Neurosurg Psychiatry. 2003;74(10):1459.

12. Buzzi MG, Cologno D, Formisano R, Caltagirone C. Hypnic headache responsive to indomethacin: second Italian case. Funct Neurol. 2005;20(2):85–7.
13. Caminero AB, Martín J, Del Río MS. Secondary hypnic headache or symptomatic nocturnal hipertensión? Cephalalgia. 2010;30(9):1137–9.
14. Caminero-Rodríguez AB, Pareja JA. Bases anatómicas y neuroquímicas que explican la frecuente asociación de las cefaleas con el sueño: el paradigma de la cefalea hípnica. Rev Neurol. 2008;47(6):314–20.
15. Capo G, Esposito A. Hypnic headache. A new Italian case with a good response to pizotifene and melatonin (abstract). Proceedings of 10th congress of the international headache society, 2001 Jun 29 to Jul 3; New York, EUA. Cephalalgia. 2001;21(4):505–6.
16. Capuano A, Vollono C, Rubino M, Mei D, Cali C, De Angelis A, et al. Hypnic headache: actigraphic and polysomnographic study of a case. Cephalalgia. 2005;25(6):466–9.
17. Casucci G, d'Onofrio F, Torelli P. Rare primary headaches: clinical insights. Neurol Sci. 2004;25(3):77–83.
18. Casucci G. Chronic short-lasting headaches: clinical features and differential diagnosis. Neurol Sci. 2003;24(2):101–7.
19. Centonze V, D'Amico D, Usai S, Causarano V, Bassi A, Bussone G. First Italian case of hypnic headache, with literature review and discussion of nosology. Cephalalgia. 2001;21(1):71–4.
20. Cerminara C, Compagnone E, Coniglio A, Margiotta M, Curatolo P, Villa MP, et al. Hypnic headache in children. Cephalalgia. 2011;31(16):1673–6.
21. Ceronie B, Green F, Cockerell OC. Acoustic neuroma presenting as a hypnic headache. BMJ Case Rep. 2021;14(3):e235830.
22. Cohen AS, Kaube H. Rare nocturnal headaches. Curr Opin Neurol. 2004;17(3):295–9.
23. Cugini P, Granata M, Strano S, Ferrucci A, Ciavarella GM, Di Palma L, et al. Nocturnal headache-hypertension syndrome: a chronobiologic disorder. Chronobiol Int. 1992;9(4):310–3.
24. Daroff RB. Hypnics headaches. Cephalalgia. 1998;18(3):123–4.
25. De Simone R, Marano E, Ranieri A, Bonavita V. Hypnic headaches: an update. Neurol Sci. 2006;27(2):144–8.
26. Diener HC, Obermann M, Holle D. Hypnic headache: clinical course and treatment. Curr Treat Options Neurol. 2012;14(1):15–26.
27. Dissanayake KP, Wanniarachchi DP, Ranawaka UK. Case report of hypnic headache: a rare headache disorder with nocturnal symptoms. BMC Res Notes. 2017;10(1):318.
28. Dodick DW, Eross EJ, Parish JM, Silber M. Clinical, anatomical, and physiologic relationship between sleep and headache. Headache. 2003;43(3):282–92.
29. Dodick DW, Jones JM, Capobianco DJ. Hypnic headache: another indomethacin-responsive headache syndrome? Headache. 2000;40(10):830–5.
30. Dodick DW, Mosek AC, Campbell JK. The hypnic ('alarm clock') headache syndrome. Cephalalgia. 1998;18(3):152–6.
31. Dodick DW. Hypnic headache. Reply to Dr Ravishankar Cephalalgia. 1998;18(10):712–3.
32. Dodick DW. Polysomnography in hypnic headache syndrome. Headache. 2000;40(9):748–52.
33. Dolezil D, Mavrokordatos C. Hypnic headache- a rare primary headache disorder with very good response to indomethacin. Neuro Endocrinol Lett. 2012;33(6):597–9.
34. Dolso P, Merlino G, Fratticci L, Canesin R, Valiante G, Coccolo D, et al. Non-REM hypnic headache: a circadian disorder? A clinical and polysomnography Cephalalgia. 2006;27(1):83–6.
35. Domitrz I. Hypnic headache as a primary short-lasting night headache: a report of two cases. Neurol Neurochir Pol. 2005;39(1):77–9.
36. Donnet A, Lantéri-Minet M. A consecutive series of 22 cases of hypnic headache in France. Cephalalgia. 2009;29(9):928–34.
37. Eccles MJ, Gutowski NJ. Precipitation of long duration hypnic headaches after ACE inhibitor withdrawal. J Neurol. 2007;254(11):1597–8.

38. Eliasson JH, Scher AI, Buse DC, Tietjen G, Lipton RB, Launer LJ, et al. The prevalence of hypnic headache in Iceland. Cephalalgia. 2020;40(8):863–5.
39. Escudero Martínez I, González-Oria C, Bernal Sánchez-Arjona M, Jiménez Hernández MD. Description of series of 10 patients with hypnic headache: discussion of the diagnostic criteria. Neurologia. 2015;30(4):195–200.
40. Evans RW, Dodick DW, Schwedt TJ. The headaches that awaken us. Headache. 2006;46(4):678–81.
41. Evers S, Goadsby PJ. Hypnic headache. Pract Neurol. 2005;5(3):144–9.
42. Evers S, Goadsby PJ. Hypnic headache: clinical features, pathophysiology, and treatment. Neurology. 2003;60(6):905–9.
43. Evers S, Rahmann A, Schwaag S, Lüdermann P, Husstedt IW. Hypnic headache – the first German cases including polysomnography. Cephalalgia. 2003;23(1):20–3.
44. Fantini J, Granato A, Zorzon M, Manganotti P. Case report: coexistence of SUNCT and hypnic headache in the same patient. Headache. 2016;56(9):1503–6.
45. Fonseca M, Teotónio P, Fonseca AC. An unsuspected cause of hypnic-like headache. J Neurol. 2016;264(2):404–6.
46. Forbes RB. Hypnic headache – your definitive guide. Northern Ireland: Forbes Neurology Services Ltd; 2013.
47. Fortes YML, Erudilho E, Silva TS, Souza WPO, Silva-Néto RP. Secondary hypnic headache: a literature review in the last 34 years. Headache Medicine. 2022;13(3):163–6.
48. Fowler MV, Capobianco DJ, Dodick DW. Headache in the elderly. Semin Pain Med. 2004;2(2):123–8.
49. Freeman WD, Brazis TW, Capobianco DJ, et al. Hypnic headache and intracranial hypotension. In: Proceedings of 46th Annual Scientific Meeting American Headache Society, 2004 Jun 10–13; Vancouver, British Columbia. Headache. 2004;44(5):498.
50. Fukuhara Y, Takeshima T, Ishizaki K, Burioka N, Nakashima K. Three Japanese cases of hypnic headache. Rinsho Shinkeigaku. 2006;46(2):148–53.
51. Garza I, Oas KH. Symptomatic hypnic headache secondary to a nonfunctioning pituitary macroadenoma. Headache. 2009;49(3):470–2.
52. Garza I, Swanson J. Successful preventive therapy in hypnic headache using hypnotics: a case report. Cephalalgia. 2007;27(9):1080–1.
53. Ghiotto N, Sances G, Di Lorenzo G, Trucco M, Loi M, Sandrini G, et al. Report of eight new cases of hypnic headache and mini-review of the literature. Funct Neurol. 2002;17(4):211–9.
54. Gil-Gouveia R, Goadsby PJ. Secondary hypnic headache. J Neurol. 2007;254(5):646–54.
55. Goadsby PJ, Lipton RB. A review of paroxysmal hemicranias, SUNCT syndrome and other short-lasting headaches with autonomic feature, including new cases. Brain. 1997;120(1):193–209.
56. Godoy JM. Remission of hypnic headache associated with idiopathic cyclic edema with the use of aminaphtone. Open Neurol J. 2010;4:90–1.
57. Gould JD, Silberstein SD. Unilateral hypnic headache: a case study. Neurology. 1997;49(6):1749–51.
58. Grosberg BM, Lipton RB, Solomon S, Ballaban-Gil K. Hypnic headache in childhood? A case report Cephalalgia. 2004;25(1):68–70.
59. Guido M, Specchio LM. Successful treatment of hypnic headache with topiramate: a case report. Headache. 2006;46(7):1205–6.
60. Holle D, Gaul C, Krebs S, Naegel S, Diener H-C, Kaube H, et al. Nociceptive blink reflex and pain-related evoked potentials in hypnic headache. Cephalalgia. 2011;31(11):1181–8.
61. Holle D, Naegel S, Gaul C, Krebs S, Gizewski ER, Diener HC, et al. Structural and functional changes in hypnic headache [abstract]. Cephalalgia. 2009;29(1):1–166.
62. Holle D, Naegel S, Krebs S, Gaul C, Gizewski E, Diener HC, et al. Hypothalamic gray matter volume loss in hypnic headache. Ann Neurol. 2010;69(3):533–9.
63. Holle D, Naegel S, Krebs S, Katsarava Z, Diener HC, Gaul C, et al. Clinical characteristics and therapeutic options in hypnic headache. Cephalalgia. 2010;30(12):1435–42.

64. Holle D, Naegel S, Obermann M. Hypnic headache. Cephalalgia. 2013;33(16):1349–57.
65. Holle D, Naegel S, Obermann M. Pathophysiology of hypnic headache. Cephalalgia. 2014;34(10):806–12.
66. Holle D, Obermann M. Hypnic headache and caffeine. Expert Rev Neurother. 2012;12(9):1125–32.
67. Holle D, Wessendorf TE, Zaremba S, Naegel S, Diener HC, Katsarava Z, et al. Serial polysomnography in hypnic headache. Cephalalgia. 2011;31(3):286–90.
68. Ivañez V, Soler R, Barreiro P. Hypnic headache syndrome: a case with good response to indomethacin. Cephalalgia. 1998;18(4):225–6.
69. Jennum P, Jensen R. Sleep and headache. Sleep Med Rev. 2002;6(6):471–9.
70. Jiménez-Caballero PE, Gámez-Leyva G, Gómez M, Casado-Naranjo I. Descripción de una serie de casos de cefalea hípnica. Diferenciación entre sexos Rev Neurol. 2012;54(6):332–6.
71. Karlovasitou A, Avdelidi E, Andriopoulou G, Baloyannis S. Transient hypnic headache syndrome in a patient with bipolar disorder after the withdrawal of long-term lithium treatment: a case report. Cephalalgia. 2008;29(4):484–6.
72. Kerr E, Hewitt R, Gleadhill I. Benign headache in the elderly – a case report of hypnic headache. Ulster Med J. 2006;75(2):158–9.
73. Kesserwani H. Hypnic headache responds to topiramate: a case report and a review of mechanisms of action of therapeutic agents. Cureus. 2021;13(3):e13790.
74. Klimek A, Sklodowski P, Night headache. Report of 2 cases. Neurol Neurochir Pol. 1999;33(5):49–54.
75. Kocasoy-Orhan E, Kayrak-Ertas N, Orhan KS, Ertas M. Hypnic headache syndrome: excessive periodic limb movements in polysomnography. Agri. 2004;16(4):28–30.
76. Lanteri-Minet M, Donnet A. Hypnic headache. Curr Pain Headache Rep. 2010;14(4):309–15.
77. Lanteri-Minet M. Hypnic headache. Headache. 2014;54(9):1556–9.
78. Liang JF, Fuh JL, Yu HY, Hsu CY, Wang SJ. Clinical features, polysomnography and outcome in patients with hypnic headache. Cephalalgia. 2008;28(3):209–15.
79. Liang JF, Wang SJ. Hypnic headache: a review of clinical features, therapeutic options and outcomes. Cephalalgia. 2014;34(10):795–805.
80. Lisoto C, Mainardi F, Maggioni F, Zanchin G. Episodic hypnic headache? Cephalalgia. 2004;24(8):681–5.
81. Lisotto C, Maggioni F, Mainardi F, Zanchin G. Caffeine efficacy in hypnic headache syndrome. Cephalalgia. 2000;20(4):332.
82. Lisotto C, Rossi P, Tassorelli C, Ferrante E, Nappi G. Focus on therapy of hypnic headache. J Headache Pain. 2010;11(4):349–54.
83. Lucchesi LM, Speciali JG, Santos-Silva R, Taddei JA, Tufik S, Bittencourt LR. Nocturnal awakening with headache and its relationship with sleep disorders in a population-based sample of adult inhabitants of São Paulo City. Brazil Cephalalgia. 2010;30(12):1477–85.
84. Manni R, Sances G, Terzaghi M, Ghiotto N, Nappi G. Hypnic headache: PSG evidence of both REM-and NREM-related attacks. Neurology. 2004;62(8):1411–3.
85. Manzoni GC, Torelli P. International headache society classification: new proposals about chronic headache. Neurol Sci. 2003;24(2):86–9.
86. Marrone LCP, Trentin S, Oliveira FM, Marrone ACH. Cefaleia hípnica em adulto jovem – Relato de caso. Rev Bras Neurol. 2010;46(1):31–3.
87. Martins IP, Gouveia RG. Hypnic headache and travel across time zones: a case report. Cephalalgia. 2001;21(9):928–31.
88. Marziniak M, Voss J, Evers S. Hypnic headache successfully treated with botulinum toxin type a. Cephalalgia. 2007;27(9):1082–4.
89. Mitsikostas DD, Vikelis M, Viskos A. Refractory chronic headache associated with obstructive sleep apnoea syndrome. Cephalalgia. 2008;28(2):139–43.
90. Molina-Arjona JA, Jiménez-Jiménez FJ, Vela-Bueno A, Tallón-Barranco A. Hypnic headache associated with stage 3 slow wave sleep. Headache. 2000;40(9):753–4.

91. Moon HS, Chung CS, Hong SB, Kim YB, Chung PW. A case of symptomatic hypnic headache syndrome. Cephalalgia. 2006;26(1):81–3.
92. Morales F. Síndrome de cefalea hípnica. Revisión Rev Soc Esp Dolor. 1999;6(5):363–7.
93. Morales-Asín F, Mauri JA, Iñiguez C, Espada F, Mostacero E. The hypnic headache syndrome: report of three new cases. Cephalalgia. 1998;18(3):157–8.
94. Moreira IM, Mendonça T, Monteiro JP, Santos E. Hypnic headache and basilar artery dolichoectasia. Neurologist. 2015;20(6):106–7.
95. Mosek A, Dodick DW. The hypnic headache syndrome: Mayo Clinic experience (Abstract). Proceedings of 8th Congress of the International Headache Society, 1997 Jun 10–14; Amsterdam, Germany. Cephalalgia. 1997;17(3):312.
96. Mulero P, Guerrero-Peral AL, Cortijo E, Jabary NS, Herrero-Velázquez S, Miranda S, et al. Cefalea hípnica: características de una serie de 13 nuevos casos y propuesta de modificación de los criterios diagnósticos. Rev Neurol. 2012;54(3):129–36.
97. Mullally WJ, Hall KE. Hypnic headache secondary to haemangioblastoma of the cerebellum. Cephalalgia. 2010;30(7):887–9.
98. Naegel S, Huhn JI, Gaul C, Diener HC, Obermann M, Holle D. No pattern alteration in single nocturnal melatonin secretion in patients with hypnic headache: a case-control study. Headache. 2017;57(4):648–53.
99. Newman LC, Lipton RB, Solomon S. Hypnic headaches. Headache. 1990;30(4):236.
100. Newman LC, Lipton RB, Solomon S. The hypnic headache syndrome: a benign headache disorder of the elderly. Neurology. 1990;40(12):1904–5.
101. Obermann M, Holle D. Hypnic headache. Expert Rev Neurother. 2010;10(9):1391–7.
102. Ouahmane Y, Mounach J, Satte A, Zerhouni A, Ouhabi H. Hypnic headache: response to lamotrigine in two cases. Cephalalgia. 2012;32(8):645–8.
103. Pascual J. Other primary headaches. Neurol Clin. 2009;27(2):557–71.
104. Patel S. Hypnic headache: a review of 2012 publications. Curr Pain Headache Rep. 2013;17(7):346.
105. Patsouros N, Laloux P, Ossemann M. Hypnic headache: a case report with polysomnography. Acta Neurol Belg. 2004;104(1):37–40.
106. Peatfield RC, Mendoza ND. Posterior fossa meningioma presenting as hypnic headache. Headache. 2003;43(9):1007–8.
107. Peng H, Wang L, He B, Giudice M, Zhang L, Zhao ZX. Hypnic headache responsive to sodium ferulate in 2 new cases. Clin J Pain. 2013;29(1):89–91.
108. Pérez Hernández A, Gómez OE. Influenza a virus: a possible trigger factor for hypnic headache? Neurologia. 2015;32(1):67–8.
109. Perez-Martinez DA, Berbel-Garcia A, Puente-Muñoz AI, Saiz-Diaz RA, de Toledo-Heras M, Porta-Etessam J, et al. Hypnic headache: a new case. Rev Neurol. 1999;28(9):883–4.
110. Peters N, Lorenzl S, Fischereder J, Bötzel K, Straube A. Hypnic headache: a case presentation including polysomnography. Cephalalgia. 2006;26(1):84–6.
111. Pinessi L, Rainero I, Cicolin A, Zibetti M, Gentile S, Mutani R. Hypnic headache syndrome: association of the attacks with REM sleep. Cephalalgia. 2003;23(2):150–4.
112. Pinto CAR, Fragoso YD, Souza Carvalho D, Gabbai AA. Hypnic headache syndrome: clinical aspects of eight patients in Brazil. Cephalalgia. 2002;22(10):824–7.
113. Pinto CAR, Fragoso YD, Souza Carvalho D, Gabbai AA. Síndrome da cefaleia hípnica: aspectos clínicos de 16 pacientes. Rev Neurociênc. 2003;11(1):46–51.
114. Pinto CAR, Fragoso YD, Souza CD. Síndrome da cefaléia hípnica: aspectos clínicos de 16 pacientes. Migrâneas e Cefaleias. 2003;6(1):17–8.
115. Pinto CAR, Fragoso YD, Souza CD. Síndrome da cefaléia hípnica: estudo polissonográfico de 9 pacientes. Migrâneas e Cefaleias. 2003;6(1):15–6.
116. Porta-Etessam J, Muñiz S, Cuadrado ML, González-García N, Orviz A, Abarrategui B, et al. Successful treatment of hypnic headache syndrome with flunarizine. J Neurol Neurosci. 2013;(4)1:2.

117. Porta-Etessam J, Pérez-Martínez DA, Martínez-Salio A, Berbel-García A, Gordo R. Successful treatment of hypnic headache syndrome with flunarizine (Abstract). Proceedings of 8th Headache Congress of the European Headache Federation, 2006 Apr 26–29; Valencia, Spain. J Headache Pain. 2006;7(1):56.
118. Porta-Etessam JP, García-Morales I, Di Capua D, García-Cobos R. A patient with primary sexual headache associated with hypnic headaches. J Headache Pain. 2009;10(2):135.
119. Prakash S, Dahbi AS. Relapsing remitting hypnic headache responsive to indomethacin in an adolescent: a case report. J Headache Pain. 2008;9(6):393–5.
120. Puca F, Prudenzano MP, Savarese M, Genco S. Headache and sleep: clinical and therapeutical aspects. J Headache Pain. 2004;5(2):123–7.
121. Queiroz LP, Coral LC. The hypnic headache syndrome – A case report (Abstract). Proceedings of 8th Congress of the International Headache Society, 1997 Jun 10–14; Amsterdam, Germany. Cephalalgia. 1997;17(3):303.
122. Rains JC, Poceta JS. Sleep and headache. Curr Treat Options Neurol. 2010;12(1):1–15.
123. Ravishankar K. Hypnic headache syndrome. Cephalalgia. 1998;18(6):358–9.
124. Rehmann R, Tegenthoff M, Zimmer C, Stude P. Case report of an alleviation of pain symptoms in hypnic headache via greater occipital nerve block. Cephalalgia. 2017;37(10):998–1000.
125. Relja G, Zorzon M, Locatelli L, Carraro N, Antonello RM, Cazzato G. Hypnic headache: rapid and long-lasting response to prednisone in two new cases. Cephalalgia. 2002;22(2):157–9.
126. Ruiz M, Mulero P, Pedraza MI, de la Cruz C, Rodríguez C, Muñoz I, et al. From wakefulness to sleep: migraine and hypnic headache association in a series of 23 patients. Headache. 2015;55(1):167–73.
127. Sandrini G, Tassorelli C, Ghiotto N, Nappi G. Uncommon primary headaches. Curr Opin Neurol. 2006;19(3):299–304.
128. Scagni P, Pagliero R. Hypnic in childhood: a new report. J Paediatr Child Health. 2008;44(1–2):83–4.
129. Schürks M, Kastrup O, Diener HC. Triptan responsive hypnic headache? Eur J Neurol. 2006;13(6):666–72.
130. Seidel S, Zeitlhofer J, Wöber C. First Austrian case of hypnic headache: serial polysomnography and blood pressure monitoring in treatment with indomethacin. Cephalalgia. 2008;28(10):1086–90.
131. Sibon I, Ghorayeb I, Henry P. Successful treatment of hypnic headache syndrome with acetazolamide. Neurology. 2003;61(8):1157–8.
132. Silva-Néto RP, Roesler CP, Raffaelli E Jr. Nocturnal headache, nightmares and lithium. Migrâneas Cefaleias. 2008;11(1):14–6.
133. Silva Néto RP, Almeida KJ. Lithium-responsive headaches. Headache Medicine. 2010;1(1):25–8.
134. Silva-Néto R. Cefaleias noturnas. In: Silva-Néto R, editor. Cefaleia – aspectos históricos e tópicos relevantes. Teresina: Halley; 2013. p. 139–44.
135. Silva-Néto RP, Bernardino SN. Ambulatory blood pressure monitoring in patient with hypnic headache: a case study. Headache. 2013;53(7):1157–8.
136. Silva-Néto RP, Almeida KJ. Hypnic headache: a descriptive study of 25 new cases in Brazil. J Neurol Sci. 2014;338(1–2):166–8.
137. Silva-Néto RP, Almeida KJ. Hypnic headache in childhood: a literature review. J Neurol Sci. 2015;356(1–2):45–8.
138. Silva-Néto RP, Sousa-Santos PEM, Peres MFP. Hypnic headache: a review of 348 cases published from 1988 to 2018. J Neurol Sci. 2019;401:103–9.
139. Silva-Néto RP, Soares AA, Peres MFP. Hypnic headache due to hypoglycemia: a case report. Headache. 2019;59(8):1370–3.
140. Silva-Néto. Cefaleia hípnica: Dores que vem pelo sono. Nova Aliança: Teresina; 2019.
141. Silva-Néto RP, Souza WPO, Krymchantowski AG, Jevoux C, Krymchantowski AV. Cefaleia hípnica: diagnóstico e tratamento. In: Valença MM, editor. Cefaleia, vol. 1. Advance in Science: Recife; 2022.

142. Skobieranda FG, Lee TG, Solomon GD. The hypnic headache syndrome: six additional patients (abstract). Proceedings of 8th congress of the international headache society, 1997 Jun 10-14; Amsterdam, Germany. Cephalalgia. 1997;17(3):304–5.
143. Son BC, Yang SH, Hong JT, Lee SW. Occipital nerve stimulation for medically refractory hypnic headache. Neuromodulation. 2012;15(4):381–6.
144. Swick TJ. The neurology of sleep. Neurol Clin. 2015;23(4):9671–89.
145. Tariq N, Estemalik E, Vij B, Kriegler JS, Tepper SJ, Stillman MJ. Long-term outcomes and clinical characteristics of hypnic headache syndrome: 40 patients series from a tertiary referral center. Headache. 2016;56(4):717–24.
146. Trucco M, Maggioni F, Badino R, Zanchin G. Hypnic headache syndrome: report of a new Italian case. Cephalalgia. 2000;20(4):312.
147. Ulrich K, Gunreben B, Lang E, Sitti R, Griessinger N. Pregabalin in the therapy of hypnic headache. Cephalalgia. 2006;26(8):1031–2.
148. Valentinis L, Tuniz F, Mucchiut M, Vindigni M, Skrap M, Bergonzi P, et al. Hypnic headache secondary to a growth hormone-secreting pituitary tumour. Cephalalgia. 2008;29(1):82–4.
149. Vieira-Dias M, Esperança P. Hypnic headache: a report of four cases. Rev Neurol. 2002;34(10):950–1.
150. Vieira-Dias M, Esperança P. Hypnic headache: report of two cases. Headache. 2001;41(7):726–7.
151. Zanchin G, Lisotto C, Maggioni F. The hypnic headache syndrome: the first description of an Italian case. J Headache Pain. 2000;1(1):60.
152. Zhang Y, Wang C, Chen Y, Wang R, Lian Y. Hypnic headache with dopaminergic neuron dysfunction: new insight from a rare case. Pain Med. 2019;20(8):1639–42.

Index

R. Silva-Néto, D. Holle-Lee, *Hypnic Headache*,
https://doi.org/10.1007/978-3-031-32263-1

MIX
Papier aus verantwortungsvollen Quellen
Paper from responsible sources
FSC® C105338

If you have any concerns about our products,
you can contact us on
ProductSafety@springernature.com

In case Publisher is established outside the EU,
the EU authorized representative is:
Springer Nature Customer Service Center GmbH
Europaplatz 3, 69115 Heidelberg, Germany

Printed by Libri Plureos GmbH
in Hamburg, Germany